SPECIAL ISSUE ON WOMEN'S HEALTH

GENDER-BASED VIOLENCE
IN THE WESTERN PACIFIC REGION:
A HIDDEN EPIDEMIC?

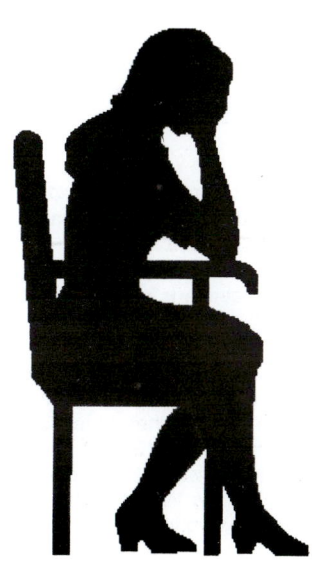

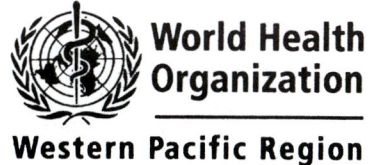

WHO Library Cataloguing in Publication Data

Gender-based violence in the Western Pacific Region : a hidden epidemic?

(Special issue on women's health)

1. Violence. 2. Domestic violence. 3. Battered women. 4. Pregnant women. 5. Sex offenses. 6. China. 7. Philippines

ISBN 92 9061 226 3   (NLM Classification: WA 309)

© World Health Organization 2006

All rights reserved.

The designations employed and the presentation of the material in this publication do not imply the expression of any opinion whatsoever on the part of the World Health Organization concerning the legal status of any country, territory, city or area, or of its authorities, or concerning the delimitation of its frontiers or boundaries. Dotted lines on maps represent approximate border lines for which there may not yet be full agreement.

The mention of specific companies or of certain manufacturers' products does not imply that they are endorsed or recommended by the World Health Organization in preference to others of a similar nature that are not mentioned. Errors and omissions excepted, the names of proprietary products are distinguished by initial capital letters.

The World Health Organization does not warrant that the information contained in this publication is complete and correct and shall not be liable for any damages incurred as a result of its use.

Publications of the World Health Organization can be obtained from WHO Press, World Health Organization, 20 Avenue Appia, 1211 Geneva 27, Switzerland (tel: +41 22 791 2476; fax: +41 22 791 4857; email: bookorders@who.int). Requests for permission to reproduce WHO publications, in part or in whole, or to translate them – whether for sale or for noncommercial distribution – should be addressed to Publications, at the above address (fax: +41 22 791 4806; Email: permissions@who.int). For WHO Western Pacific Regional Publications, request for permission to reproduce should be addressed to Publications Office, World Health Organization, Regional Office for the Western Pacific, P.O. Box 2932, 1000, Manila, Philippines, Fax. No. (632) 521-1036, Email: publications@wpro.who.int

TABLE OF CONTENTS

Acknowledgements 4

Preface 5

Part 1. Introduction 7

Part 2. Suicidal behaviour among women of child-bearing 13
age: Report of an investigative study in Longde County,
Ningxia Hui Autonomous Region, China

Part 3. Domestic violence against pregnant women and its 55
impact: A survey in Northern China

Part 4. Medico-legal and health services for victims of 113
sexual violence: A situational analysis in the Philippines

Acknowledgements

WHO is grateful to the institutions who have contributed during the development of this document, and to the committed individuals whose experiences were reflected in this document. To the interviewers for collecting relevant information and data.

Preface

In 1996, the World Health Assembly declared violence "a leading worldwide public health problem"[1] and Murray and Lopez[2] reported that the global burden of injury from violence falls disproportionately on females of all ages. It is this nexus between violence as a key health issue and as a gender issue that is explored in this publication.

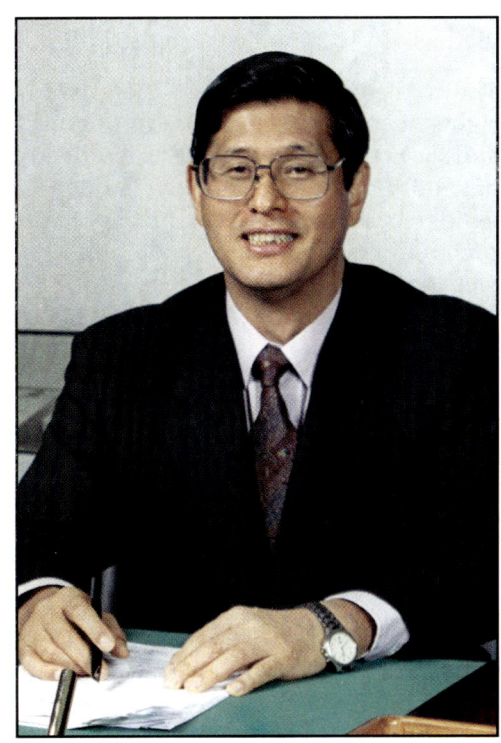

The 2005 WHO Multi-country Study on Women's Health and Domestic Violence Against Women[3] found that abused women were twice as likely as non-abused women to have poor health and physical and mental problems, even years after the violent attacks have ceased. The symptoms included suicidal thoughts and attempts, mental distress and physical symptoms like pain, dizziness and vaginal discharge. They also had increased risk of sexually transmitted infections, including HIV. Prevalence rates for domestic violence were higher than expected. In particular, in pregnant women, prevalence rates of violence by an intimate partner, usually the father of the unborn child, were found to be 4% to 12%. However, there are still data gaps for the Western Pacific Region, as only two countries from the Region were represented in the Multi-country Study.

The two countries from the Region which were included in the WHO Study had the lowest (Japan) and the highest (Samoa) prevalence rates for gender-based violence, including violence against pregnant women. The alarmingly high rates of non-partner physical and/or sexual gender-based violence (62% lifetime prevalence) and partner physical and/or sexual gender-based violence (46.1% lifetime prevalence) in the only country which has been subjected to a total population study, Samoa, suggests the urgent need to establish reliable data from large-scale prevalence studies in other countries in the Region to see if they too have a 'hidden' epidemic.

In line with the recognition of the WHO Western Pacific Regional Office that gender-based violence is a major public health issue, it has put together this publication to showcase some of the important epidemiological and evaluation research on the topic that is being conducted in other parts of the Region. The three studies contained in this volume provide complementary data for the Western Pacific Region to support the mission of the Multi-country Study.

The first two studies provide much needed epidemiological data on two aspects of gender-based violence in China, self-directed violence and intimate partner abuse. The third provides a comprehensive evaluation of services for abused women in the Philippines. In the Introduction, Liz Eckermann, from Deakin University in Australia, provides a situational analysis of gender-based violence internationally, regionally and nationally, identifies where the three studies fit into WHO's typology of violence[4] and points to the commonalities between the three studies.

---

[1] (WHA49.25)
[2] Murray C, Lopez A. (1996) *The Global Burden of Disease, Vol.1.* Harvard, Harvard School of Public Health, 1996.
[3] *WHO Multi-country Study on Women's Health and Domestic Violence Against Women.* Geneva, World Health Organization, 2005.
[4] *World report on violence and health.* Geneva, World Health Organization, 2002.

In the first study, researchers Wang Yan, Huang Fei, Shi Ling and An Lin, from the School of Public Health, Peking University, report on an in-depth qualitative survey of suicidal behaviour among women of child-bearing age in Longde County in the Ningxia Hui Autonomous Region of China. In the second study, Guo Sufang, Wu Jiuling, Qu Chuanyan and Yan Renying, from Peking University and the Ministry of Health, provide findings from an extensive survey of intimate partner abuse against pregnant women and recent parity women in northern China. In the final study, Pagaduan-Lopez, Pagaduan, Bazaar, Salud, Rodriguez and Pareno undertake a situational analysis of medico-legal and health services for victims of sexual violence in the Philippines.

The challenge is to convert the growing recognition of gender-based violence as "a serious human rights abuse" as well as "an important public health problem that concerns all sectors" [5] into action and services. All three projects involved action research, whereby training and education about aspects of gender-based violence is integral to the research process. For example, in the study on prevalence of gender-based violence against pregnant and recent parity women in northern China, the health practitioners who helped gather the epidemiological data attended a one-week workshop where they were trained on research methods as well as gender-based violence theories, diagnosis, treatment, referral and prevention strategies.

The dearth of prevalence research relates very much to the difficulties of undertaking such studies. Definitions of domestic violence are slippery, it is still a taboo and a 'private' and 'shameful' issue in many cultural contexts, and gender-based violence is such an integral part of so many cultural traditions that it is often 'normalized' and dismissed as 'just part of life' [6]. These seemingly insurmountable barriers have not deterred the three groups of researchers whose work appears in this volume. They have undertaken systematic quantitative and qualitative research on gender-based violence which provides much needed data to inform service provision as well as health promotion and violence prevention initiatives in the Region.

Shigeru Omi, MD, Ph.D.
Regional Director

---

[5] *Op cit.* Ref 3:1.
[6] *Op cit.* Ref 4.

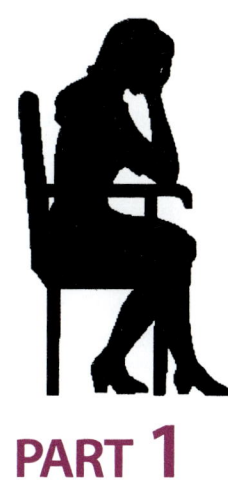

PART 1

INTRODUCTION

GENDER-BASED VIOLENCE IN THE WESTERN PACIFIC REGION: A HIDDEN EPIDEMIC

VIOLENCE AS A MAJOR PUBLIC HEALTH ISSUE: INTERNATIONALLY, REGIONALLY AND NATIONALLY

The World Development Report 1993[1] identified violence against women as a major contributor to the burden of ill-health internationally in terms of "female morbidity and mortality, leading to psychological trauma and depression, injuries, sexually transmitted diseases, suicide and murder". Those conclusions were reinforced in 1996 by Murray and Lopez[2] who found that, although injury from violence of all types was a major contributor to the global burden of disease for both sexes, that burden falls disproportionately on females of all ages. The health dimensions of violence were confirmed in 1996 when the World Health Assembly declared violence a "leading public health problem"[3]. In 1998, the WHO Regional Office for the Western Pacific conducted a review of domestic violence in the thirty-seven countries and areas of the Region[4] and came to the same conclusions.

Comparing prevalence rates for different countries across the Western Pacific Region was difficult because of varying definitions of what constitutes domestic violence, cultural taboos and the normalization of violence in many areas, all leading to a lack of political will and the consequent absence of reliable data. However, very conservative estimates were made suggesting that prevalence rates and lifetime prevalence rates for domestic physical violence against women in the countries and areas of the Western Pacific Region were between 5.8% and 61%, and for sexual abuse between 4% and 50%. In most cases, those figures represent serious underreporting and in many cases de facto indicators of abuse were used (such as suicide rates and divorce rates) given the reluctance of survivors, perpetrators and authorities to provide reliable direct data.

As part of its ten-year review of the implementation of the recommendations of the 1994 International Conference on Population and Development (ICPD,1994), ARROW reviewed progress on reducing domestic violence for eight countries, four of which fall within the Western Pacific Region: Cambodia, China, Malaysia and the Philippines[5]. ARROW argued that "one of the best indicators of real change in power relations between men and women is a decrease in domestic violence and rape" yet only two of the ten countries that they reviewed, Cambodia and Malaysia, "had ever had a national prevalence survey on domestic violence"[6]. The review found that domestic violence prevalence rates had not decreased in Cambodia over the ten years since ICPD, despite government-sponsored legal and service intervention. The lifetime prevalence rate for partner violence in one town, Pursat, had climbed to 47% given that "perpetrators of sexual exploitation, trafficking and rape of women and children continue to escape legal punishment because of corruption, lack of legal protection, and ignorance of rights"[7]. In Malaysia, best estimates of spousal abuse prevalence in women over 15 years of age were around 39%[8]. In China, figures on gender-based violence were so tentative that they were not given. However gender-based negligence by parents, including malnutrition, is reported as widespread and 70% of women have "no insurance cover at all"[9]. Similarly, the statistics on domestic violence from the Philippines were too sketchy to come to any clear conclusions about progress.

Thus the three research projects presented in this volume are valuable contributions towards filling some of the epidemiological gaps in knowledge about the prevalence and incidence rates of self-inflicted and intimate partner violence in two countries of the Region, China and the Philippines, for which there are very limited data. They provide a detailed complement to the overview study conducted by WHO and discussed below.

---

[1] World Bank. *World Development Report 1993: Investing in Health*, Oxford, Oxford University Press, 1993:50.
[2] Murray C, Lopez A. *The Global Burden of Disease, Vol.1.* Harvard, Harvard School of Public Health, 1996.
[3] Resolution WHA49.25
[4] Domestic violence: A priority public health issue in the Western Pacific Region, Manila, WHO Western Pacific Regional Office, 1998.
[5] ARROW *Monitoring Ten Years of ICPD Implementation: The Way Forward to 2015: Asian Country Reports.* Kuala Lumpur, ARROW, 2005.
[6] *Ibid*: 43.
[7] *Ibid*: 359.
[8] *Ibid*: 244.
[9] *Ibid*:170.

INTRODUCTION

Since the end of the twentieth century, WHO has been conducting a multi-country in-depth study of the health effects of domestic violence against women[10]. The study has broadened the violence against women agenda on many fronts. First, the multi-country study acknowledges the "combined efforts of grass-roots and international women's organizations, international experts and committed governments" in producing "a profound transformation of public awareness" about gender-based violence[11]. Since the World Conference on Human Rights (1993), the International Conference on Population and Development (1994) and the Fourth World Conference on Women (1995), the perception of gender-based violence as purely a welfare and justice issue has changed dramatically in many quarters. Violence against women is "now widely recognized as a serious human rights abuse" as well as "an important public health problem that concerns all sectors"[12]. Second, the indicators used to measure the impact of gender-based violence have been broadened to encompass quality of life issues, as well as social indicators. Third, the WHO study has brought to the fore the importance of focusing on the ethical considerations of any research, and the impact of ethical practice on research outcomes. The informed consent, safety, privacy and confidentiality of participants are key methodological considerations. Fourth, the WHO multi-country study has started to change the terminology that we use to refer to violence against women. The term 'gender-based violence' is increasingly being used to imply that there is a theory that explains violence rather than just using descriptive terms such as 'violence against women'.

Japan and Samoa were the only countries from the Western Pacific Region included in the ten-country WHO study. Japan was chosen for its position on the low end of the violence prevalence scale and Samoa for its position towards the top of the scale, so neither country is representative of the Region as a whole. However, in Samoa the whole country was surveyed, so a comprehensive picture of various forms of violence against women can be constructed.

Of the ten countries, Japan (city location) had the lowest prevalence rates of physical abuse (13%), sexual abuse (6%) and lifetime physical and/or sexual abuse (15%) by an intimate partner, and also the lowest rates for non-partner abuse of all kinds. By contrast, Samoa had the highest rates of non-partner physical violence (62%), and non-partner sexual violence since age 15years (>10%) and high (but not the highest) rates of all forms of intimate partner abuse. While these data provide some guidelines for reform in Samoa and a benchmark for good practice in urban Japan, many gaps remain in research on gender-based violence in the Region.

Despite attempts to change terminology, challenges remain in defining exactly what it is that we are talking about when we refer to various forms of violence and abuse in establishing accurate prevalence rates and mobilizing political will for change in some countries. The projects reported in this publication take on board those challenges for two countries in the Region.

TYPOLOGY OF VIOLENCE

The three research projects reported in this issue use a shared typology to define the aspects of violence on which they are concentrating. In 1996, the World Health Assembly charged WHO with the responsibility to develop a typology of violence to encourage a shared understanding of violence and to start the process of generating research and prevention programmes. The WHO typology was first used systematically in the *World report on violence and health*[13], which identifies three broad categories of violence according to the characteristics of those committing the violent act. These are: self-directed violence, interpersonal violence and collective violence. It must be noted that the typology represents and 'ideal type' given that in the real world the boundaries between the three categories often blur and are not as discrete as the typology suggests.

---

[10] Multi-country Study on Women's Health and Domestic Violence Against Women. Geneva, World Health Organization, 2005.
[11] *Ibid*:1.
[12] *Ibid*:1.
[13] *World report on violence and health*. Geneva, World Health Organization, 2002:6.

This current special issue deals with sub-categories of the first two categories of violence as perpetrated against women: suicidal behaviour and intimate partner abuse (see Figure 1). Such abuse can be physical, sexual, or psychological or take the form of deprivation and neglect. In the case of suicidal behaviour, self-directed abuse can be the end result of sexual or other forms of abuse. Abuse often involves a combination of these forms of violence and, when systematically perpetrated against women, applying the term 'gender-based violence', alongside the typology, facilitates analysis.

In Part 2, researchers from the Department of Maternal and Child Health, Peking University, isolate as their focus the issue of suicidal behaviour among women of child-bearing age in Longde County in the Ningxia Hui Autonomous Region of China. In Part 3, still in China, Guo Sufang, Wu Jiuling, Qu Chuanyan and Yan Renying, from Peking University and the Ministry of Health, report on a survey of intimate partner abuse against pregnant women and recent parity women in the northern part of the country. In Part 4, Pagaduan-Lopez, Pagaduan, Bazaar, Salud, Rodriguez and Pareno undertake a situational analysis of medico-legal and health services for victims of sexual violence in the Philippines.

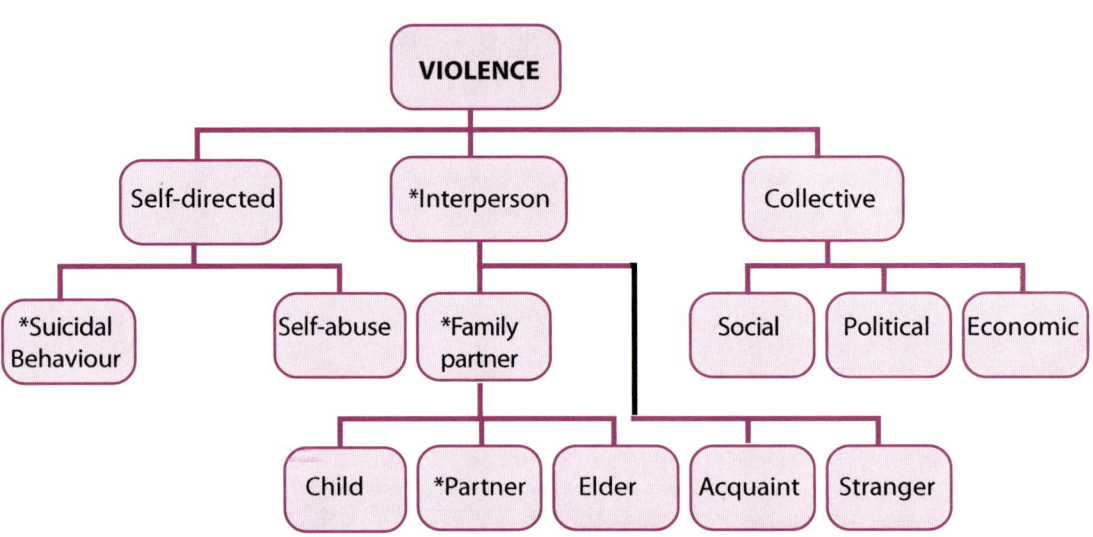

Figure 1. Typology of violence adapted from World report on violence and health, highlighting # areas covered in this volume.

COMMONALITIES BETWEEN THE THREE PROJECTS: GENDER-BASED VIOLENCE

The findings reported in Parts 2 to 4 represent three separate attempts to fill some of the knowledge gaps in our understanding of gender-based violence. Although the topics are slightly different, the aims are the same: to provide a comprehensive gender analysis of the power relationships between men and women and the impact of the abusive aspects of those relationships on the health of women, men and children, and on society as a whole. It is noteworthy that, despite the differences in focus between the three projects, the conclusions and recommendations dovetail into each other. This suggests that some deep-seated forces are at play in the etiology and perpetuation of both self-inflicted and interpersonal violence, and in the resistance on the part of authorities and functionaries to implement change to prevent such violence.

The objectives of the study in Part 2, on suicidal behaviour amongst women of child-bearing age in Longde County, China, were to: identify causes, motivations and risk factors for the women, to explore prevention options and to provide evidence for agencies to act on prevention. The results indicate a strong gender dimension in incidence and prevalence, given that women attempt suicide at four times

INTRODUCTION

the rate of men. Family conflict emerges as the major proximal and distal cause of suicide attempts. Other factors contributing to suicide attempts include social factors such as poverty, low status in the family and community, poor education and lack of social support, and triggering factors related to family conflict and violence, although such violence also forms part of the general social backdrop for the women who attempt suicide. The major risk factors are domestic violence, depression, lack of family cohesion and negative events. The preventive measures proposed vary from practical measures, such as restricting access to mouse poison and providing appropriate counselling and support, through to more systemic recommendations, such as improving women's social standing and quality of life and educating both men and women about human rights issues.

In Part 3, Guo and colleagues investigate the prevalence of intimate partner violence before, during and after pregnancy in women in four provinces of northern China. The study examines the factors leading to violence and the consequences on the health and well-being of the mothers and their children. The study adopts a gender perspective, asking the women respondents and focus groups of men about gender roles and expectations. It also addresses the knowledge, attitudes and practices, related to intimate partner violence, of health providers in the four provinces. The results show a total prevalence rate of 12.6%, with physical abuse at 3.5%, sexual abuse 8% and psychological abuse 5.6%. Contrary to other research on violence during pregnancy, the study found that intimate partner violence decreased to 4.3% during pregnancy (9.1% before pregnancy and 8.3% after delivery). The key correlates with intimate partner violence are history of abortion, severity of depression, lifetime experience of intimate partner violence and relationship conflict/neglect/economic control. The lack of acknowledgement, on behalf of some women, most men and health care providers, that intimate partner violence constitutes serious abuse, is alarming. Most respondents 'normalized' intimate partner abuse, arguing that it is a private concern rather than a serious public health, justice and human rights issue. The recommendations put forward include urgent training of health providers on service provision, diagnosis and referral for domestic violence and gender awareness. Multisectoral cooperation is also recommended to deal with the range of agencies with a vested interest in prevention, including the police, the judiciary, social services, NGOs and human rights advocacy groups. Media and education campaigns about gender and human rights, targeted at all groups in the population, are proposed to deal with the deep-seated gender biases in the background culture of populations in northern China.

In Part 4, the theme of gendered construction of violence continues. Pagaduan-Lopez and colleagues document the structures and resources of the Philippine health sector's response to sexual violence and the process of service delivery that is provided in three sites (Manila, Sorsogon and Oriental Mindoro). The study operated at two levels, the national and provincial government level and the facility level. At the macro level the Department of Health and the National Bureau of Investigation were the sources of data. At the micro level, three data collection instruments were employed at the three sites: a facility checklist of equipment and supplies, a questionnaire for the service managers and a questionnaire for the service providers. The opinions of other interested parties, such as the police, social welfare agencies and NGOs, were also canvassed. Although there have been significant legal and service networks (including laws against marital rape, women's desks in police facilities and dedicated hospital facilities) set up throughout the Philippines to address sexual violence, the study found that the facilities are often poorly equipped and the staff undertrained, and sometimes unmotivated. Thus the quality of care for victims and perpetrators is compromised. Furthermore, the researchers found that the majority of the population still see sexual violence as a criminal justice and social concern rather than a human rights and health issue. The role of family support is integral in short- and long-term outcomes of sexual violence, but this presents a dilemma in that family members can also be perpetrators, and points to the central role of ethical considerations, especially in relation to safety, privacy and confidentiality, in provision of services for survivors of sexual abuse.

The three studies make a significant contribution to an understanding of gender-based violence in two countries of the Western Pacific Region which have not previously been researched adequately. Although tackling different parts of the violence typology (Figure 1), the three projects share key elements which make their findings comparable with the data collected for the WHO Multi-country Study. These commonalities between the three projects are reflected in the language which is increasingly being used to replace terms such as domestic violence, intimate partner violence and violence against women.

The term 'gender-based violence', which encapsulates the focus of all three projects in this special issue, contains an implicit theory about the source of the violence and allows for an analysis of both women's and men's parts in prevention.

First, they all adopt a gendered perspective of violence, acknowledging that many of the solutions to such violence involve long-term systemic changes to the way men and women relate to each other. All three projects point to the burden of tradition in maintaining unequal gender roles. They share an optimism that change is possible, not only in gender roles, but also in the popular perception that gender-based violence is merely a justice and social services problem rather than a key health and human rights issue. In fact, the authors of all three studies would concur with ARROW[14] that a reduction in gender-based violence is a key indicator of palpable change in power relationships between the sexes, which benefits the health and well-being of both men and women. Thus, all three projects have as their ultimate outcome Millennium Development Goal 3: to promote gender equality and empower women[15]. However, their recommendations go beyond the official MDG Target 4 (to eliminate gender disparity targets in primary and secondary education by 2015) to cover all aspects of life, including power relationships within families.

Second, all three research projects clearly elaborated a set of ethical protocols and considerations in gathering data which, not only protected the integrity and safety of the participants, but also ensured more reliable data, given that participants' involvement in the research was voluntary rather than being dictated (or denied) by the power of partners or other family members.

Third, all three projects broadened the indicators used to measure outcomes, beyond mortality and morbidity, to include process indicators (including equipment and service delivery) and quality of life and social indicators. The results of data gathered using such broad indicators allow for intervention at all levels, from individual therapy and rehabilitation to population-based mass media and education campaigns to reduce gender-based violence.

---

[14] *Op cit.* Ref 11:43
[15] United Nations *Millennium Development Goal Indicator Database*, New York, United Nations, 2005.

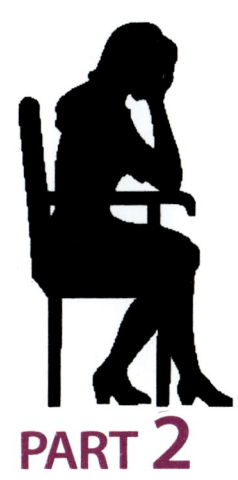

PART 2

SUICIDAL BEHAVIOUR OF WOMEN AMONG CHILD-BEARING AGE

REPORT OF AN INVESTIGATIVE STUDY IN LONGDE COUNTY,
NINGXIA HUI AUTONOMOUS REGION, CHINA

TABLE OF CONTENTS

Abstract	15
Chapter 1. Background	18
Chapter 2. Objectives	20
Chapter 3. Design and methods	20
Study site	20
Study methods	20
Study sample	20
Study content	21
Implementation and quality control	24
Chapter 4. Findings and results	25
General conditions	25
Current suicide situation	26
Risk factors for suicide	35
Attitude to suicide	42
Suicide prevention	45
Chapter 5. Discussion and conclusions	47
Discussion	47
Suggestions for prevention	51
Remaining challenges	53

Abstract

OBJECTIVES

- To identify the risk factors, including psychological, biological, family (including family violence), community and social factors, for suicidal behaviour among women of child-bearing age;
- to determine the motives for and methods of suicide, and events that may have precipitated the suicidal act;
- to investigate the availability and effectiveness of social support networks and health care facilities (governmental and nongovernmental) for preventing women's suicide; and
- to explore effective measures for prevention of and intervention on women's suicide, therefore providing scientific information and recommendations for a national strategy for suicide prevention.

METHODS

Quantitative and qualitative methods were employed to investigate women who attempted suicide in Longde County, Ningxia Hui Autonomous Region from 15 November 2001 to 14 November 2002. The methods included a hospital-based case-control study, individual in-depth interviews and focus group discussions.

RESULTS

1. Suicide attempts

A total of 47 women attempted suicide during the period investigated. Of those 47 women, 41 were of child-bearing age, five of whom died. During the same period, 14 men attempted suicide, all unsuccessfully. Ten of those men were aged 15 to 49. Therefore, for women of child-bearing age, the number of attempted suicides was 4.1 times higher than for men of equivalent age; the number of attempted suicides was 7.2 times the number of completed suicides.

2. Method

Of the 36 women of child-bearing age who survived a suicide attempt, one cut her wrist and the remaining 35 took poison. Of the 35 who took poison, 26 (74.3%) took mouse poison; 20 took poison stored at home and the other 15 bought poison just before attempting suicide.

3. Causes

The main cause of the women's suicide attempts was family conflict (72.2%). That family conflict, and the concomitant domestic violence and abuse, was mainly caused by financial difficulties. Other reasons included unhappy marriages and life difficulties.

4. Social attitude to suicide

A few people questioned said they thought suicidal behaviour was justified, especially when a woman was suffering from an untreatable disease or had done something 'immoral'. However, the majority of people held negative attitudes towards suicide. They thought it would not solve any problems, but could have adverse effects on individuals, families and society, especially on children. The majority of people were sympathetic towards suicide victims and the families involved, and suggested that they would like to keep contact with them as usual.

5. Motivation

Three types of motivation for women's suicidal behaviour were evident. These were:

Impulse. Some women attempted suicide on impulse after experiencing 'special' events. Among the investigated 36 women who attempted suicide, 27 women (75.0%) regretted attempting suicide after being rescued.

Threat. Some women hoped to threaten others by attempting suicide, as a means of asking for more respect from their husbands or families.

Escape. Some women could find no better way to deal with their difficulties than death, so they attempted suicide as a way to solve their problems or escape from difficulties.

6. Risk factors for suicide

6.1. Domestic violence:

The women who attempted suicide were more likely to experience domestic violence than the control group of women. The proportions "having been beaten by husband" and "being beaten by husband in the last year" among those women who attempted suicide were significantly higher than among the control group, indicating that domestic violence is one of the risk factors for women's suicide. The main reason given for domestic violence were family conflict and financial difficulties.

6.2. Depression:

There was a significant difference in the incidence of depression between the case group and the control group. The cases were more likely to have feelings of guilt, self-punishment, self-abhorrence and suicidal intention than the controls.

6.3. Family cohesion:

Sixty-nine women out of 72 (36 pairs of cases and controls) participated in the investigation on family cohesion and adaptability. The three women who did not participate were given average scores. A paired t-test showed that cohesion in the control group's families was higher than in the case group's families.

6.4. Negative life event:

A significant difference was found between the case and the control groups in scores on negative life events. The women who attempted suicide were more likely to have experienced negative life events, including poor marital relationships, marital separations of longer than one month, financial difficulties and having debts of over 500 Yuan (US$62).

6.5. Multivariate statistics analysis

Univariate predictors with a p value < 0.05 were employed in multivariate conditional logistic regression analysis. Two variables, "being beaten by husband in last year" and "suicidal intention", entered into the model when statistical significance was defined as pd"0.05. The other two variables, "having been beaten by husband" and "negative life events", were significant risk factors for suicide attempts at the level of 0.1.

7. Factors contributing to women's suicide attempts

Questionnaire data from the women who had attempted suicide and the controls, as well as in-depth interview data from informant and focus group discussions, were used to identify the factors contributing to the suicide attempts.

As shown in Figure 1, women living in poor rural environments work hard at domestic chores and farming all their lives, suffer from low status in society and often experience violence within their families. Lacking available legal mechanisms and social support systems, such women are more inclined to feel helpless and depressed when being abused, and may therefore choose suicide as a way to resolve their difficulties and relieve their intense sadness.

Figure 1 illustrates the etiological chain of events leading to suicide attempts for many women. This combination of contributing factors has been demonstrated in many studies of suicidal behaviour, and this research reinforces those findings. Women's suicide is the result of interaction between environmental, family and individual factors. Poverty and women's low status are the source of conflict. Family conflict and the accompanying domestic violence are triggering factors, and easy access to lethal poisons is the facilitating factor for suicide.

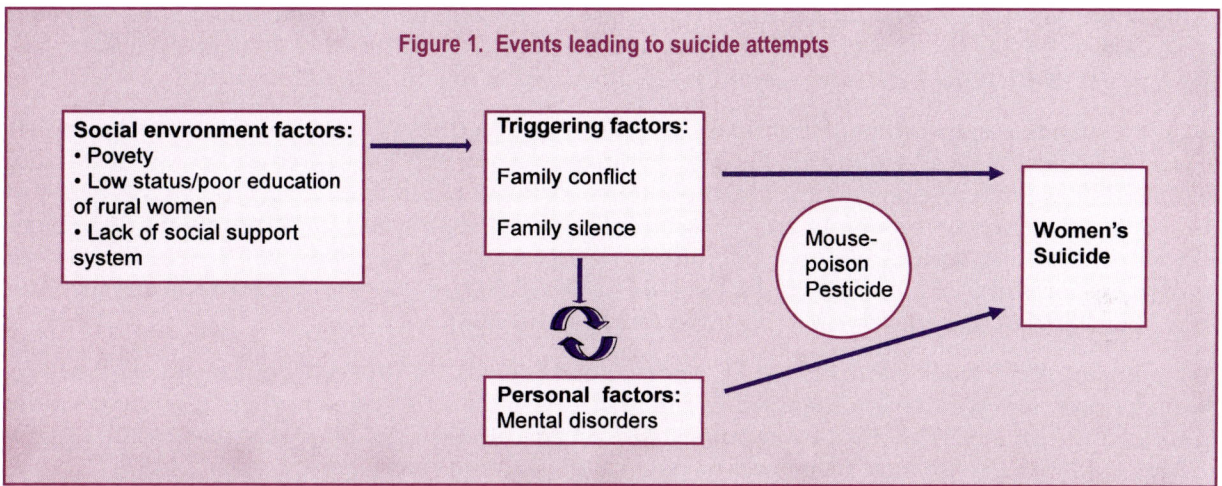

8. Preventive measures

Some preventive measures aimed at reducing the identified risk factors are proposed. They include restricting access to the means of suicide, improving women's quality of life, improving women's positions in their families and society, eliminating family violence, paying particular attention to women who have attempted suicide, establishing suicide prevention centres and implementing integrated prevention programmes.

CHAPTER 1.
BACKGROUND

Suicide is the intentional self-inflicting act of ending one's own life[1]. Suicidal behaviour is a phenomenon that has many determinants, and is closely associated with physiological, psychological, family and social factors. Due to its universality and the human cost, suicidal behaviour is attracting increasing attention from governments, agencies and researchers.

Suicide is a major public health problem worldwide. In many industrial countries, suicide stands among the ten leading causes of death; for young people, suicide is currently the third leading cause of death[2]. Globally, deaths due to suicide have increased by 60% in the past 45 years, from 10.1 per 100 000 in 1950 to 16 per 100 000 in 1995. According to data from 97 countries and regions, in 2000, suicide was estimated to have caused one million deaths. This translates to one person dying due to suicide every 40 seconds[3]. The number of attempted suicides is about 10-20 times that of deaths caused by suicide[4].

In China, suicide is a disturbing public health problem and a significant source of mortality. According to the 1998 National Health Statistics, the suicide rate was 20 per 100 000, with the rates varying across regions[5]. For example, the highest suicide rate among women of child-bearing age in 1996 was found in rural areas of moderate economic growth, where the adjusted suicide mortality rate was 35.97 per 100 000. The second highest was in economically disadvantaged rural areas (23.72 per 100 000), the third in economically advantaged rural areas (16.78 per 100 000), the fourth in middle and small cities (10.97 per 100 000), and the lowest in big cities (5.20 per 100 000).

According to WHO health statistics for 44 countries and regions for 1994, the highest suicide rate was found among rural women in China. Furthermore, China is the only country where more women die from suicide than men. The suicide rate among women aged 15-34 is double that of men, while in most countries, four to five times as many men as women die through suicide.

A comparison of different countries shows that, for each reproductive age period, the highest suicide rate is found among women of rural China. There is also a peak in the suicide rate for women aged 15-34 in urban areas[6]. Suicide has been a major cause of death for this age group in China since 1990. In 1998, suicide was the leading cause of death for the overall population of 15-34 year-olds. More specifically, it was the leading cause of death among rural women aged 15-34 and urban women aged 15-24; the second leading cause of death among urban women aged 25-34 and among rural men aged 15-24; the third leading cause among rural men aged 25-34; and the fourth leading cause among urban men aged 15-34[7,8].

Previous studies have identified poisoning (mouse poison or pesticide) as the most common method of committing suicide among rural women in China, accounting for 68% to 92% of all female suicides in rural areas[9,10,11]. The main causes of women's suicides are interpersonal conflicts, family problems, financial difficulties, mental distress and physical disease [12,13,14,15].

---

[1] Li Hongzheng, Lei Meiying. Study progress on suicidal behaviour of foreign soldiers. *Foreign Medical Sciences*, Psychiatry Section, 2000, 27(3):140-143.
[2] Liu Huaqing£¬Li Xianyun. Study status quo and trend of suicidal behaviour. *Foreign Medical Sciences*, Psychiatry Section, 1996; 23(2): 81-86.
[3] Xu Wenqing. Health promotion intervention on suicide prevention. *Chinese Health Education Journal*, 2001; 17(7): 446.
[4] Desjarlais R. *et al. World mental health: problems and priorities in low-income countries.* New York, Oxford University Press, 1995.
[5] Op cit. Ref 3.
[6] Yang Junfeng£¬An Ling£¬Wang Shaoxian. Fatal suicide analysis of Chinese reproductive-aged women. *Population Study.* 24£¨6£©.
[7] Op cit. Ref 3..
[8] Li Xianyun, Fei Lipeng. Fatal suicide causes analysis of Chinese reproductive-aged population in 1998. China *Public Health*, 2001, 17(7) :658-660.
[9] Wan Junfeng. Epidemiological analysis on 1107 cases of suicide. *Anhui Journal of Preventive Medicine*, 2000; 6(2):119.
[10] Tang Xiaolan, Jiao Jiege, Gao Hongsheng. Epidemiological survey on the attempted suicides, in Qionghai city, Hannan province. *Chinese Journal of Disease Control & Prevention*, 2001, 5(3):204-206.
[11] Xu Huilan *et al.* Epidemiological study on the suicidal elders in cities and townships, Hunan province. *Chinese Mental Health Journal*, 2000, 14(2):121-124.
[12] Op cit. Ref 3.
[13] Yin Hong et al. Suicidal causes analysis on inhabitants in Liangping county in 1990~1992. *Chinese Mental Health Journal*, 1999, 13(2): 113.
[14] Wang Faxin *et al.* Correlative factors analysis of attempted suicides. *Chinese Behavior Medical Science*, 2002, 11(3): 288-29.
[15] Wang Jiahua. Case reports on 179 attempted suicides. *Chinese Mental Health Journal*, 1998, 12(6): 378-379.

Suicide is not only a major cause of death, but also a mirror which reflects serious public health and social problems. The suicide rate is highest for rural women of child-bearing age, which is a major burden on women's lives and health and has serious social and economic costs for fragile economies. Compounding the tragedy of loss of life are the many more women who attempt suicide and are saved by improved medical intervention. Therefore, the number of suicide deaths represents only a small portion of the problem. Such a high suicide attempt rate among women reflects profound social problems, which have severe impacts on women's physical and mental health.

A wide range of disciplines have regarded suicidal behaviour and suicide prevention as significant topics. A comprehensive review of existing studies[16,17,18,19,20,21,22,23,24,25,28,27,28,29,30,31,32] reveals that most of them have been aimed at young people, persons with mental disorders, homosexuals and the elderly, while few studies have targeted women of child-bearing age. Most existing suicide research uses clinic-based case studies that focus on suicides or attempted suicides admitted to hospitals, while community-based studies are rare. Those studies that are community-based are restricted to describing the characteristics of suicide and are less developed in terms of identification of the social, economic, cultural, environmental and other factors contributing to the suicide attempts. Much still remains to be learnt in that area.

This study is conducted, therefore, to identify the causes, motives and risk factors concerning suicidal behaviour of women of child-bearing age in China. It also explores and develops feasible approaches to suicide prevention among women, and provides scientific information for the establishment of national strategies to prevent suicide and, ultimately, to protect and improve women's health.

---

[16] *Op cit.* **Ref 8.**
[17] *Op cit.* **Ref 9.**
[18] *Op cit.*.**Ref 10.**
[19] *Op cit.* **Ref 11.**
[20] *Op cit.* **Ref 13.**
[21] *Op cit.* **Ref 14.**
[22] *Op cit.* **Ref 15.**
[23] Liu Lianzhong, Xiao Shuiyuan. Follow-up study on attempted suicides. *Chinese Mental Health Journal*, 2002, 16(4): 253-256.
[24] Zhao Zhixiu. Psychological analysis and strategies on 103 cases of suicides. *Journal of Mathematical Medicine*, 2001, 14(3): 247.
[25] Zhang Rongqin. Psychological survey analysis on 425 cases of suicides of 2001. *Henan Medical Information*, 2001, 9(18):4-5.
[26] Li Xianyun etc. The case-control study on the risk factors of attempted suicide. *Chinese Journal of Epidemiology*, 2001, 22(4):281-283.
[27] Eggert LL, *et al.* Preliminary effects of brief school-based prevention approaches for reducing youth suicide-risk behaviors, depression, and drug involvement. *Journal of Child and Adolescent Psychiatric Nursing*, 2002, Apr-Jun, 15(2): 48-64.
[28] Paul JP, *et al.* Suicide attempts among gay and bisexual men: lifetime prevalence and antecedents. *American Journal of Public Health*, 2002 Aug, 92(8): 1338-45.
[29] Conwell Y, *et al.* Access to firearms and risk for suicide in middle-aged and older adults. *American Journal of Geriatric Psychiatry*, 2002 Jul-Aug, 10(4): 407-16.
[30] Preuss UW, *et al.* Comparison of 3190 alcohol-dependent individuals with and without suicide attempts. *Alcohol Clin. Exp. Res.* 2002 Apr, 26(4): 471-7.
[31] Conwell Y, *et al.* Suicide in elders. *Annals of the New York Academy of Sciences*, 2001 Apr 932: 132-47; discussion 147-50.
[32] Horowitz LM, *et al.* Detecting suicide risk in a pediatric emergency department: development of a brief screening tool. *Pediatrics*, 2001 May, 107(5): 1133-7

CHAPTER 2. OBJECTIVES

The objectives of the Study on Suicidal Behaviour among Women of Child-bearing Age, conducted in Longde County, Ningxia Hui Autonomous Region, China were:

(1) to identify the risk factors, including the psychological, biological, family (including family violence), community and social factors, for suicidal behaviour among women of child-bearing age;

(2) to determine the motives for and methods of suicide, and events that may have precipitated suicidal acts;

(3) to investigate the availability and effectiveness of social support networks and health care facilities (governmental and nongovernmental) for preventing women's suicide; and

(4) to explore effective measures for prevention of and intervention on women's suicide, therefore providing scientific information and recommendations for a national strategy on suicide prevention.

CHAPTER 3. DESIGN AND METHODS

STUDY SITE

Longde County, Ningxia Hui Autonomous Region.

STUDY METHODS

The study used quantitative and qualitative methods, including a case-control study (questionnaire investigation conducted with cases and controls), registration data for suicides, individual in-depth interviews, focus group discussions and field observations.

STUDY SAMPLE

1. **Case-control study**

    1.1. Cases (Women of child-bearing age who had attempted suicide)

    Criteria: All women of child-bearing age who attempted suicide and were admitted to the county hospital or township hospitals from 15 November 2001 to 14 November 2002.

    1.2. Controls

    Criteria: Female patients who were admitted to the same hospitals due to acute diseases other than suicide (within one week of admission of the controls).

Matching terms: 1:1 match was adopted. The controls had the same gender and marital status and similar careers as the cases, but had no previous suicide histories. The controls were aged 15-49 years and there was no more than three years difference between the ages of the case and the control in each matched pair.

1.3 Sample size

There were 36 cases and 36 controls.

2. Registration of completed suicide cases

Completed suicide cases were the women admitted to the county hospital or township hospitals from 15 November 2001 to 14 November 2002, and who died due to suicide.

3. Focus group discussions

During the first month of the investigation (November-December 2001), three townships were randomly selected from those where the suicide cases lived. From each of the three townships, one village was selected, giving a total of three villages as sample villages. From each sample village, male and female villagers were selected and divided into six groups as follows:

- Group A: Single males aged 15 to 24 years;
- Group B: Single females aged 15 to 24 years;
- Group C: Married males aged 20 to 34 years;
- Group D: Married females aged 20 to 34 years;
- Group E: Married males aged 35 to 49 years;
- Group F: Married females aged 35 to 49 years.

Sample size: 18 focus group discussions were held with those chosen from the three sample villages, with 6-10 participants in each group.

4. Individual in-depth interviews

Individual in-depth interviews were conducted with:

- women who had attempted suicide: 16 women who attempted suicide from 15 November 2001 to 20 April 2002;
- officials of the County Health Bureau: two persons, including the Director and the Chief of the Maternal and Child Health Project Office;
- officials of the County Women's Federation: two persons, including the Director and an assistant;
- physicians of the County Hospital: two persons, including the Dean of the Hospital and the Director of the Emergency Ward; and
- deans of the township hospitals: three deans from the sample township hospitals.

STUDY CONTENT

A questionnaire was administered to 36 women (cases) who had attempted suicide, as well as to the 36 controls.

1. Women's health questionnaires

Questionnaire A was used by the case group and Questionnaire B by the control group. The two questionnaires were the same in the first seven parts, and differed in the eighth part only.

Part 1 Individual characteristics: name, age, educational level, occupation, marital status, religious belief.

Part 2 Family characteristics: family structure, family income, parents' condition.

Part 3 Marriage condition: degree of satisfaction with marriage, family violence.

Part 4 Individual recent condition: The Beck Depression Inventory (BDI) was used to evaluate the degree of depression of cases and controls.

> The Beck Depression Inventory (BDI) is a 21-item test with each of the 21 items corresponding to a specific category of depressive symptom or attitude. Each category consists of a graded series of four self-evaluative statements. The statements are rank-ordered and weighted to reflect the range of severity of the symptom from neutral to maximum severity. Numerical values of zero, one, two or three are assigned to indicate the degree of severity. The sum of the 21-item scores can measure the degree of depression: a score of 4 or lower would be considered normal or would signify a slight disturbance; 5-13, mild depression; 14-20, moderate depression; 21 or higher, severe depression.

Part 5 Family cohesion: Family Adaptability and Cohesion Evaluation Scales II - Chinese Version (FACES II-CV) were adopted to assess the relationship between family members.

> FACES II-CV contains a total of 30 items, each item having a 5-point score choice: Never =1, Occasionally =2, Sometimes =3, Often =4, Always =5.
>
> Cohesion is the degree to which there is emotional bonding between and among family members. Adaptability is the extent to which the family system is flexible and able to change its roles and relationships in response to stress. The cohesion and adaptability scores are calculated according to the following formulae:
>
> The cohesion score = 36+I~1+I~5+I~7+I~11+I~13+I~17+I~21+I~23+I~25+I~27+I~30-I~3-I~9-I~19-I~29
>
> The adaptability score = 12+I~2+I~4+I~6+I~8+I~10+I~12+I~14+I~16+I~18+I~20+I~22+I~26-I~24-I~28
>
> (Note: I~X corresponds to the score of the Xth item.)

Part 6 Life event: The Life Event Scale (LES) was used to evaluate, both quantitatively and qualitatively, the mental pressure and impact of specific life events on women.

> LES consists of 48 items on three aspects in a checklist format. The first is family life (28 terms), the second is working and study life (13 terms), and the third is other events in social life (7 terms). There are also two blank terms to fill in for those events not listed on the form but experienced by interviewees.
>
> Methods of calculating the magnitude of events:
>
> Magnitude of a given life event= the degree of mental stress × duration of the event × frequency of the event.
>
> Magnitude of positive life events= Sum of magnitude of all positive life events.
>
> Magnitude of negative life events= Sum of magnitude of all negative life events.
>
> Total magnitude of life events= Magnitude of positive life events+Magnitude of negative life events.

Part 7 Overall condition evaluation: the interviewees' general opinions about individuals and families.

Part 8 (Questionnaires A and B had different content):

For Questionnaire A: motivations and reasons for suicide, and the method used.

For Questionnaire B: A suicide attitude questionnaire was used to investigate people's opinions on and attitudes towards suicide. The suicide attitude questionnaire was composed of 29 terms in four sections: attitude towards suicidal behaviour, attitude towards person committing suicide, attitude towards the family involved, and attitude towards euthanasia. The scores of each section were summed up and averaged. Then the attitude was evaluated based on the average score: ≤ 2.5 would be considered holding a positive, affirmative and tolerant attitude; 2.6~3.4, holding an ambivalent or indifferent attitude; ≥ 3.5, a negative, opposing and prejudiced attitude.

2. Registration data on suicide

There were two sets of registration forms. The first set was for all suicide events (completed and attempted), including the general circumstances of the suicides and the outcomes; the second was used for the completed suicides, to learn the characteristics of the women involved (age, occupation, etc), and the time and method of suicide.

3. Individual in-depth interviews

There were three outlines for different interviewees:

3.1 Outline 1

Object: women of child-bearing age who had attempted suicide.

Content:

- Causes and the whole process of suicide, and social and cultural circumstances of the incident.
- Opinion on suicidal behaviour among women of child-bearing age.
- Availability and adequacy of social support and health services provided by the local organizations to prevent suicide.
- Feasible measures to prevent the women of child-bearing age from attempting suicide.

3.2 Outline 2

Object: Officials of the Health Bureau and the Women's Federation.

Content:

- Social and cultural circumstances of women's suicidal behaviour.
- Availability and utilization of social support and health services for suicide prevention.
- Future plans, measures and restricting factors to prevent women from attempting suicide.
- Suggestions for preventing suicide among women of reproductive age.

3.3 Outline 3

Object: doctors and deans of hospitals.

Content:

- Relationship between women's suicidal behaviour and their social circumstances.
- Opinions on suicidal behaviour among women of reproductive age.
- Availability and utilization of social support and health services for suicide prevention.
- Future measures for preventing women from attempting suicide.

4. Focus group discussions

Object: Villagers of different age groups.

Content:

- Reasons for women's suicide attempts and the social, historical or cultural background.
- Attitudes and opinions regarding women's suicidal behaviour.
- Availability of social support and services for preventing women's suicide.
- Needs and future measures for suicide prevention.

5. Field observation and interview

Object: Chiefs of the organizations that provide services to prevent women's suicide attempts.

Content:

- Current services provided by the organizations for suicide prevention.
- Difficulties in suicide prevention, suggestions and future measures.

IMPLEMENTATION AND QUALITY CONTROL

1. Study design

The research plan and protocol, including all the questionnaires and interview outlines, were thoroughly discussed by the research team and invited experts, and were tested through exploratory fieldwork.

2. Research team

The data collection team consisted of three faculty members and one graduate student from the Department of Maternal and Child Health, Peking University (in-depth interviews and focus group discussions), two doctors from the emergency ward of the County Hospital and two doctors from each township hospital (registration forms for suicides and investigation of women who had attempted suicide).

The data collection team worked under the supervision of a graduate student from the Department of Maternal and Child Health, Peking University. Officials from the County Health Bureau and the Dean of the County Hospital facilitated all the work.

3. Quality control

The data collection team was trained by the graduate student from Peking University, under the supervision of Professor An Lin from Peking University.

All the questionnaires were checked by the investigators on the day when they were completed and then double-checked by the supervisor every two to three days. Any errors were corrected and the missing items re-investigated.

The data were checked for out-of-range responses and the logistical relationship between the variables.

4. Consistency rate

The consistency rate of data on 16 attempted suicides during the period from 15 November 2001 to 20 April 20 2002 was 98.3%.

Chapter 4.
FINDINGS AND RESULTS

GENERAL CONDITIONS

1. Economic conditions in Longde County

Longde County is a mountainous area in the western part of Six-Turn Mountains, in the south of Ningxia province. The total population is 210 000, of which 95% are of Han nationality. Like most of the counties in the west of China, Longde County is economically underdeveloped and has been designated a 'national poverty county'. Traditional agriculture is the primary source of income and the average annual per capita income is about 1000~1100 Yuan or approximately US$ 124-136 (official data).

A local public health official described the county's economic status in the following terms:

> *Our county is one of the national poverty counties. The average annual income per capita is less than 1000 Yuan. Even in the county centre (downtown), the income is only between 1500 and 1600, and unemployed workers have only 200-300 Yuan every month. People are not satisfied with their incomes, especially farmers; their incomes are quite low and they have a lot of financial difficulties.*

Faced with such financial difficulties, more and more male adults are swarming into the cities to make a living. This has a negative impact on women and families, since the wives and the elderly have to bear the whole responsibility of household chores and farm work.

2. The family role of women

2.1 Housework

Most rural women have to take responsibility for all the housework (including child care, cooking, laundering, dish washing) as well the farm work (including feeding and tending the cattle). The stress of performing dual roles and the heavy work is exhausting, and psychosomatic diseases are common.

2.2 Farming

In addition to housework and tending cattle, rural women have to do other farm work, such as planting, weeding and harvesting. Only heavy physical labour, such as hauling fertilizer and wheat, is done by men. When their husbands leave the area to make a living, women have to take over all the farm work. Only in the busy season do their husbands come back to help them.

2.3 Raising children

Rural women bear most of the responsibility of raising children, such as feeding, washing, dressing and providing study support. Fathers do not spend much time on child care, except for taking a sick child to hospital when necessary.

The following comments are from interviews with villagers regarding the division of labour in the family:

Men do the heavy labour and women do the trivial. What women do is boring and petty; however, women have to get up early and go to bed late.

Women work longer than men. Their work is trivial and time-consuming.

Men do the heavy work, such as transporting fertilizer or hauling wheat. Sometimes women also come to help them. However, work such as raising children, cooking, washing, raising cattle etc is done by women alone.

In conclusion, rural women are under onerous physical and psychological pressure. Often their work is boring and repetitive and, when their husbands travel to the cities to seek work, they are left with dual domestic and farming roles. During the interviews, many women expressed the wish that they had been born men instead of women.

CURRENT SUICIDE SITUATION

1. Suicide in Longde County

Longde County has a population of 210 000. In the past few years, there have been 170 to 180 suicide attempts per year, mainly by women of child-bearing age. A total of 47 women attempted suicide in the year investigated: 41 of them were women of child-bearing age, of whom five died. During the same period, 14 men attempted suicide and all survived (10 of them were aged 15 to 49 years). The number of suicide attempts by women of child-bearing age was 4.1 times greater than that by men; the number of attempted suicides was 7.2 times the number of completed suicides.

2. Attempted suicides among women of child-bearing age

2.1 Demographic characteristics

Among the 36 attempted suicides, most of them were married, of Han nationality, farmers and uneducated, or at best educated to primary-school level (see Table 1).

Table 1. Demographic characteristics of women who attempted suicide from 15 November 2001 to 14 November 2002

Nationality		Marital Status		Occupation			
Han	Hui	Married	Unmarried	Farmer	Student	Teacher	Village Doctor
5	1	33	3	32	2	1	1

Educational background			
Illiterate	Primary School	Middle School	High School
16	11	16	3

The age distribution of women who attempted suicide is shown in Table 2. The median age was 32.5 years. Nearly half (47%) of all attempted suicides occurred between the ages of 25 and 34 years.

Table 2. Age distribution of women who attempted suicide from 15 November 2001 to 14 November 2002

Age	Frequency	Percentage
15~	04	11.1
20~	02	05.6
25~	07	19.4
30~	10	27.8
35~	03	08.3
40~	05	13.9
45~49	05	13.9
Total	36	100.0

2.2 Suicide methods and sources of poison

As can be seen from Table 3, only one woman attempted suicide by cutting her wrists. The other 35 women attempted suicide by poisoning: 26 cases (74.3%) took mouse poison; 20 took poisons stored at home and the other 15 bought poison just before attempting suicide.

Table 3. Type of poison taken by women who attempted suicide from 15 November 2001 to 14 November 2002

Type	Frequency	Percentage
Mouse poison	26	74.3
Pesticide	04	11.4
Overdosing with sleeping pills	04	11.4
Others	1	2.9
Total	35	100.0

It was learnt from the interviews that mouse poison could be bought easily in markets, and most families had prepared mouse poison for killing mice. This facilitated women's impulsive and non-impulsive suicide attempts.

The following are excerpts from interview records:

Many years ago, hanging was the most common method of suicide, but now taking poison has become the most frequent in our county, especially mouse poison. The reason is obvious - mouse poison is very easy to get. Why? Because mice are rampant in rural areas, so that raticides are sold in the market, everywhere, in fact in almost every village. Although we have made many efforts to manage the sale of mouse poison, it is still not under legislative control. A government management system hasn't been established yet to control the sale of poisonous substances. We have sellers from all over the country, especially from Henan province.

Public health official

Taking poison is the most common method used for women's suicides......Because pesticide and rate poison are easily to access and purchase. Sometimes you can find lethal pesticide at home.

Another public health official

Most women commit suicide by taking poison, and it accounts for approximately 90% of suicides.......The most frequently used mouse poison is called 'Dead in a second', and this is sold by private traders. The second most common poison is phosphoric zinc, which is also a kind of lethal toxic mouse poison.

Doctor

It is impossible to jump down from a high place because there are no high buildings here. But raticide can be found at home, and it is convenient.

What can be obtained easily will be chosen, so it's more likely for our rural women to take mouse poison."

Villagers

2.3 Location of suicide attempt and weather conditions

A total of 35 women attempted suicide at home and one at an unknown place. Fifteen cases committed suicide in cloudy weather, and the other 21 on sunny days.

2.4 Motivation for suicide

Among the 36 attempted suicides, 24 (66.7%) women said that they had really wanted to die when attempting suicide; 27 (75.0%) women had regretted the suicide attempt when they were revived. The majority of the women had attempted suicide on impulse; 72% of them had spent less than five hours from having a suicidal idea to attempting suicide. Only one woman had contemplated it for 90 days (see Table 4).

Table 4. Length of time from suicide idea to action

Duration	Frequency	Percentage
<1 Hour	14	38.9
1~4 Hours	12	33.3
24~25 Hours	05	13.9
48~72 Hours	04	11.1
90 Days	01	02.8
Total	36	100.0

The interviews revealed three types of motivation for suicide among rural women: impulse, threat and escape.

Impulse

Most women had attempted suicide on impulse, in temporary despair or anger, and without friends' or relatives' advice. They had not thought seriously about the outcomes when they attempted suicide. They were so angry after conflicts with their husbands or families that they had ceased to think rationally.

As can be seen from the individual in-depth interviews with women who had attempted suicide, **family conflict was a major** factor:

After he (husband) beat me, I became very angry and lost my mind. I cannot recall exactly what happened to me. I just felt in despair. Life was hopeless. I thought it for a while, then drank the poison......

Siew

I felt mad and angry when my husband beat me. I ran to the gate and saw the poison on the windowsill. I took it without thinking. But I could only drink a little before my husband took it away and sent me to hospital......

Kah Po

I quarreled with my mother-in-law for more than one hour. She (mother-in-law) stayed in her room, and I was in my room. I lost my mind and took the pesticide, but I couldn't swallow it down, so I stopped. At that time, nothing was in my mind, it was empty.

Sun

Threat

Some women had attempted suicide as a way to threaten their families, usually after quarrelling. Unlike suicide attempts made on impulse, they had some other intentions when attempting suicide, for example, they had wanted their families (especially their husbands) to follow their advice, or give them more status in the family. They did not actually wish to die.

The following are parts of individual in-depth interviews with women who attempted suicide to threaten their husbands or families:

I attempted suicide only once, never before. Last December, we quarreled over a little thing about our children. After quarreling, I wanted to walk away from him for a while, but he stopped me and was going to beat me. I felt insulted and got rather mad, then I took up the bottle (mouse poison). I intended to show him that I was taking the poison. I was just intending to scare him, because of his bad temper and heavy beating. I didn't swallow down the poison, but only placed the bottle in my mouth, He of course saw it, and then he sent me to hospital......

Leung

I just intended to scare him at that moment. I didn't want to die in fact. My husband sent me to hospital, and I told the doctor that I didn't take the poison. I just put the paper, which wrapped the raticide, against my mouth, but I didn't actually take it. I wanted him to be scared and not beat me any more afterwards...... At that time, although I felt hopeless, I still did not want to die, I just wanted to teach him a lesson. Since then, we haven't quarreled anymore.

Lo

Escape

Some women had attempted suicide just because they had thought there was no way to continue life as it was. They had felt they were unable to resolve their difficulties and relieve their intense sadness. They had regarded suicide as a means of freeing themselves. Those women mostly belonged to disadvantaged populations in rural areas. They usually had low social positions, not being well educated or well informed. When faced with difficulties, they had not known where to seek help. Thus they had selected suicide as a way to end their unbearable pain.

The following are parts of interviews with women who attempted suicide as a means of escape:

At that moment I thought the poison could settle everything, but I feel regretful now. I have to sustain the pain caused by the suicide. Since the day I took poison, I have suffered from a stomachache all the time, but I do not have the money to see the doctor or pay for medicine......

Tze

After quarrelling with me, he (my husband) went out. I flew into a fury and did not want to live. I felt life was hopeless and meaningless. I worked hard all year, but couldn't save any money.......

Wan

My father-in-law is an old fogey, always wanting to control everything, and often beating us. He (my husband) is obedient, but I couldn't sustain it anymore. We have been married for 14 years, and I have always been beaten by my father-in-laws. I felt disgrace in facing others and I didn't want to live any longer. I thought of taking poison ......

Luan

2.5 Causes of suicide

The main cause of women's suicide attempts was family conflict (see Table 5). As learnt from the qualitative investigation, most family conflicts derive from financial difficulties. The villagers and local groups said that conflict usually arose in a family when money was needed urgently, and trivial family issues could trigger the fight. For example, when kids ask for tuition fees or farmers need money to buy fertilizer, people become anxious, irritated and easily involved in quarrels. Sometimes women curse their husbands' incapacity and poverty, and the men retaliate by using their fists against their wives. As a result of domestic violence, women commit suicide by taking poison in anger and despair.

However, although financial difficulties were given as the main reason for the family conflicts which lead to women's suicide attempts, other family conflicts, extramarital affairs, economic deprivation and mental illness were also causes (see Table 5).

Table 5. Causes of women's suicide attempts

Reason	Family conflict	Unhappy marriage	Financial deprivation	Jealousy/ envy	Others	Total
Frequency	26	4	1	1	4	36
Percentage	72.2	11.1	2.8	2.8	11.1	100.0

The following information was obtained from in-depth interviews with local groups and villagers:

One public health official, Yong, argued:

Women are usually at the lowest position in families. When there is a fight between a wife and her husband, between a wife and her mother-in-law, or between neighbours, the woman is not likely to get support from her family, thus she may choose suicide. Few women attempt suicide just because of poverty. They usually have other reasons, say mental illness.

Another public health official, Suan, proposed that:

In remote areas, the number of suicide attempts is very high. Why? The first reason is the women's low educational level; the second is the narrow scope and short sight, of people who don't know how to resolve their problems; the third is a lack of law consciousness; and the fourth is a lack of belief in future life, especially for rural women, who are likely to feel helpless and attempt suicide when they encounter difficulties. For example, one old woman, because her son didn't care for her, felt despair and committed suicide. The fifth reason is conflict between daughters-in-law and mothers-in-law. Most of these conflicts are temporary and won't last long. The sixth reason is long-lasting disharmony between the couple.

As for family conflict, there are many causes, such as disharmony between the couple. In urban areas, it's usually caused by the husband's unfaithfulness, extramarital affairs. But in rural areas, the main reason is family trivia. We describe the relationship between rural couples as "rice-bread wife and husband -, the better the economic status, the better the relationship, and vice versa. It is common here. The second reason is that the husband doesn't share household work or the husband indulges in gambling, and doesn't care for the family. The third reason is treating family members unequally, such as a daughter-in-law not respecting her parents-in-law, or parents-in-law abusing the daughter-in-law. Then conflicts are likely to occur.

One member of the Women' Federation, Goh, said:

In my opinion, the leading cause of women's suicide attempts is extramarital affairs. In the past we could only see 'extramarital love' in the media, we heard about 'having a second wife' from big

big cities, but now these stories are going on in our county, even in rural areas. We hear these from time to time when local women come to us for help.

Dr Wong, a physician, suggested:

Most women attempt suicide on impulse, while some of them contemplate it for some time and prepare the poison in advance. Let me think, the main reason is conflict between the couple. What causes the conflict? As I know, some money difficulty is always triggering the war. Most women attempt suicide for this reason (economic deprivation). You know, suicide is most frequent in the busy season in farming. When the family cannot continue the farming work because they cannot afford fertilizer, they get anxious and come to battle. Then the woman attempts suicide as a result. Such events are relatively rare in the slack season. Besides financial difficulty, kid's problems also cause fights in the family. For instance, a husband feels dissatisfied with the wife because she can't bear a son, then the wife becomes suicidal. This is rare, of course. Another cause is the disharmonious relationship between the couple. Their relationship breaks up and they want to get divorced. When it fails, the wife attempts suicide.

Another physician, Dr Teow, hypothesized that:

The main cause of women's suicide attempts here is poverty. In economically developed areas, maybe extramarital love is the main reason, but in our poor rural area the poor economic status is the main reason, because it can easily induce conflict between husband and wife, or between daughter-in-law and parents-in-law. The second leading reason is disharmony between the wife and her parents-in-law. The parents-in-law usually look down on and abuse their daughter-in-law. This leads to conflict between the husband and wife. As a result, the woman attempts suicide. There are also some cases due to extramarital love or disputes with parents, for example, a woman chooses a boyfriend but her family don't accept him. These are infrequent however.

In conclusion, the leading cause of suicide is family conflict; and the second is the disharmonious relationship between couples, such as extramarital love affairs. Other reasons, such as being abused by others, are relatively rare. Generally speaking, financial difficulty accounts for 60%-70% of women's suicides, marriage problems for 20%, and conflict between mother-in-law and daughter-in-law for 10%.

In individual interviews, women who had attempted suicide revealed their reasons.

At the chat time at dinner, I answered my mother-in-law back about for a little thing. It made her unhappy. After that, I was going to clean the house, but she didn't permit it. Then we had a quarrel. My husband heard the voices and came to me. He slapped me in the face without asking any reason. I felt angry and started crying. Then my mother-in-law returned to her room (next to our room) and my husband went to bed, leaving me alone in the kitchen doing the cooking. When I thought over these things, I felt unbearable anger. I started to abuse them. I thought 'You beat me, and then you go to sleep! My life is horrible; there is no reason for me to live'. This thought reminded me that there was some mouse poison left in our barn, so I went to the barn to get it. My husband followed me to the barn. I faced him, and put the wrapping paper of the poison into my mouth, but I did not actually take it. He thought I did, and sent me to hospital......

Lo

I failed my exam at school. On the way home, my classmates laughed at me and I started to quarrel with them. Other classmates tried to stop us, but it was useless because we were angry at that time. I didn't say anything to my parents when I came back home. Mum asked me to pass a cup of water to grandpa, but I didn't do it because I was still angry with my classmates. Mum blamed me for a while, and I still didn't tell her about my examination failure. After my mother turned to cooking, I started crying in my room. Crying and crying, suddenly I thought of death, so I cut my wrist with a knife. I saw blood, but not much. I was not frightened and went to call mum. Mum then sent me to hospital......

Pung

It happened because of money. One day when I bought wool for my kid, I owed the seller some money. I asked my husband to send the money to the seller. He did not agree. Then I asked him to give me the money so that I could return it to the seller, but he still didn't agree. He told me no money. I quarreled with him, blamed him, and he came to beat me. I lost my temper and cursed him. After I finished cooking, I didn't take anything but the pesticide......

Chang

We have two daughters, but are without a son. The older daughter has got married, the younger hasn't. Our son-in-law is living with us, called "Dao cha men" here. We had thought that he would support us till the end of our lives.

He came from another village. As our neighbours know, my family is the most honest in this village, but he was still very picky and always found fault. In the second year since he came to live with us, he started to make trouble. It lasted for 4-5 years. Sometimes, my husband and I didn't interfere with them, because we wanted the couple to settle their issues by themselves. However, even doing so, he did not stop making trouble at home. Sometimes we could not tolerate it and I thought of suicide. We went to village groups for help. They came to mediate between us, but to no effect. For this reason, local villagers were unwilling to visit my home.

Because of poverty, he went outside to work in the slack season. In the first ten days after he returned, things were all right, but ten days later he started making trouble, such as complaining about the cooking, and my daughter could not stop him either. He has been doing so for 4-5 years. He did some home work when he was happy, otherwise, he would go to bed. My daughter got angry, but she could not find a solution ......

Why I took the poison this time? It was due to his provocation. At the end of the year, we used to kill a pig. My daughter didn't boil the water on time because she had to lull her kid first. My son-in-law was dissatisfied and shouted at her. It was noon. As usual, we should have treated the persons who had helped us to kill the pig to lunch, but we had to delay it to the next day because of his unhappy behaviour. The next day, he was still angry and abused my daughter, from the evening when all guests left to the next morning when my husband fed the cattle. My daughter was lulling their child. I changed my clothes and then took the poison.

After doing these things, I sat on the bed and talked with my husband. I asked him to care for our younger daughter who was still single. In addition, I said "It is unlucky that you are sick, but after all, our older daughter has a child." My husband felt something was wrong with me, and asked me if I had taken something. I felt faint, so my husband sent me to hospital with the help of others......

Dang

Luan also suggested that a trivial matter had triggered her suicide attempt:

You would laugh at me if I told you because I attempted suicide just because of some little things. One day, our electric iron didn't work and my husband decided to fix it by himself. However, he connected the wrong wire and burned the iron. Then he bought a new wire, but he made the same mistake again. When I blamed him for it, he was irritated and fought back, then we moved into a fistfight. Later, he told his father that I was a shrew. His father came to me and rebuked me for it. He told his son that he would teach me a lesson the next time. The next day, my husband went to his aunt's home at 11 o'clock asking for work. At 12 o'clock, my father-in-law came to me saying that I had driven his son away from home, and he ordered me to find him. I said that I was very busy then, it was the time to feed the livestock, to care for the children from school, to prepare the lunch, as well as do some housework. I am a tailor, you know. I am very busy. I told him that I did not know where his son was. My father-in-law became angry and hit me with a stick. My face was bleeding and my arms were hit at that time, but he didn't stop beating. Therefore I fought back with a stick and blamed him, saying "you sell the evil idea!" He intended to hit me more, when my mother-in-law came and stopped us. She said some words to me and pulled my father-in-law out. They left me alone. At that time, my head was bleeding more and more, but I didn't feel panic at all, I just wrapped my head in a scarf. I felt faint and went to bed to have a sleep. Women in rural areas indeed have a lot of grievances. I was told later that my father-in-law went to the village commission complaining that I had hit him with a stick.

At 2 o'clock I awakened and found my head still bleeding, and I went to the township hospital. I was angry and in pain. As a woman living in a rural area, bearing a son is the most important. I have two kids, one girl and one boy, and everything looks fine. My kids are well, my husband is nice. We would have had a quiet life since we live independent of his parents, but my father-in-law was so traditional that he insisted on disturbing me more.

I supported the family, taking care of everything, but they still made trouble. I would have felt better if my husband had beaten me instead of my father-in-law. People who knew my father-in-law considered it his fault; those who didn't, however, blamed me. It is miserable, I want to leave home and work outside. I believe I could support myself.

On that day, when I stayed in hospital receiving fluid transfusion, I thought that my children would not be cared for well if I died. I thought of death first, but I denied this thought. I told myself "I am still young and have two kids to take care of. I shouldn't end my life, even although we are poor and my husband is weak."

But when I returned home from the hospital, my husband still hadn't come back. I cooked for my kids, but I ate nothing. I had lost my appetite. I thought of why my husband hadn't come back. I would have felt much better if he had been home and comforted me with some warm words. I thought it back and forth during the night. I thought if I could have owned more knowledge and skills, I would not have been treated like this. My husband's a coward, and I was beaten by my-father-in-law after 14 years of marriage. This deeply disgraced me. There was no reason for me to live anymore, so I decided to take poison. At 9 o'clock, the second day after I came back from the hospital, I took the mouse poison.

Goh pointed to financial issues as the trigger for her suicide attempt.

It was 3pm, Lunar January 10th (*Chinese traditional calendar*). My daughter was going to school at Yinchuan city, so I packed the bags for her. I asked my husband to prepare 800 Yuan for our daughter, but he told me there was no money left. I said that we couldn't let our daughter drop out of school even if we had to ask the bank for a loan. He said he did not want the kid to continue her school anymore because we had spent more than 5000 Yuan on her. Just at that time, my daughter came to him asking for money. He actually beat her! I went up to protect my daughter and blamed him, he started to beat me as well. My kid was crying, and I got mad. I thought that the whole family was depending on my salary completely (I am a teacher), and I worked hard for my kids. But finally I couldn't afford my kid's schooling. I suffered enough! So I took the poison, a kind of powder for killing mice, in my room while my husband was scolding my kid in another room. I started to vomit before I could swallow it down. My husband found it and sent me to hospital. I was discharged on the second day.

Thus financial factors, family conflicts and often trivial events can trigger suicide attempts. However, usually there has been a build up of stress and tension over some time and the minor event becomes the 'last straw'. Those in touch with the stressed woman need skill to sense her high level of stress and despair before the precipitating event.

2.6 Symptoms exhibited before suicide

Most women exhibit mood disorders before attempting suicide, including pessimism, sadness and irritability (see Table 6). A total of 20 women had felt pessimistic and sad before their suicide attempts. They had felt apathetic and a loss of hope. Eight women had been irritable before their suicide attempts, showing emotional instability. Family members, friends and neighbours should be alert to such signs and symptoms. Particular attention should be paid to those who are experiencing serious sadness, distress or pessimism.

Table 6. Symptoms exhibited before suicide

Symptoms	Frequency	Percentage
Asymptomatic	7	19.4
Sadness	20	55.6
Guilt	1	2.8
Irritability	8	22.2
Total	36	100.0

The women who had attempted suicide revealed the following in in-depth interviews:

Fong described the despair and sense of abandonment she felt prior to her suicide attempt:

I felt rather angry after being beaten by my husband. I lay in bed alone for two days, nobody caring about me. I wanted to leave home, but it's impossible, I would worry about my kids. But I could not bear his bad temper. Life is hopeless, I am so sad.

Sun, described a mixture of anger and despair:

I quarreled with my mother-in-law for more than one hour. I was almost mad at that time, caring about nothing, not even my kids. So I took the pesticide.

Chang described a feeling of intense pain leading up to her suicide attempt:

After quarreling with my husband, I felt unbearable pain. I am useless, know nothing, only make a mess. He could find a better one if I died.

2.7 Difficulties in life

Although half of the women who had attempted suicide did not record any difficulties in their lives in their questionnaire responses (see Table 7), it was learnt from in-depth individual interviews that most of them had experienced a variety of difficulties, especially economic deprivation.

Table 7. Life difficulties for women who attempted suicide

Difficulties	Frequency	Percentage (%)
None	16	44.5
Financial difficulties	9	25.0
Health problems	3	8.3
Financial and health problems	3	8.3
Marital problems	4	11.1
Learning difficulties	1	2.8
Total	36	100.0

Many rural women suffer various difficulties, but there are no specific organizations to help them out of those difficulties. Although there are Women's Federations and village commissions, they are not familiar, accessible or helpful to many women. The women interviewed said they always felt hopeless and were unable to see alternative solutions to their problems.

They reported the following as the troubles most frequently experienced:

The kid is ill and nobody takes care of him. My husband goes out to make a living. I worry about my kid but I don't have the money to send him to hospital.

I have been sick for a long time, but we are poor, so I have to endure the pain. I still have to do the housework and help with the farming.

We are poor, so my husband goes out to make money, leaving me alone to take care of everything at home, caring for the elderly and feeding the kids. I am exhausted.

Women have to do everything, housework and farming. We still have to feed cattle and cook for kids. We do both men's and women's jobs.

We can't eat well, dress well; we don't even have more clothes to change. Taxes, utilities, everything needs money, but we don't have money.

Thus, lack of access to a variety of resources – financial, social support, health services – are key background factors predisposing women to attempt suicide. When a trigger factor emerges which undermines their resilience to constant poverty and lack of social capital, they may attempt to end their miserable lives.

2.8 History of suicide

Only one case out of 36 left a note before attempting suicide. Only four had attempted suicide before, all by self- poisoning. After being rescued, the majority of the women who had attempted suicide said that they would never attempt suicide again in the future. However, some women said they did not exclude the possibility of attempting suicide when facing similar problems at a later stage. As one woman said:

It's hard to say now. If the problem still exists and can't be resolved, I might attempt suicide again.

RISK FACTORS FOR SUICIDE

1. Educational level, religious beliefs and beliefs about death

A comparison between cases and controls indicated that women's educational level, religious beliefs and beliefs about death had no significant effect on their likelihood to attempt suicide (see Table 8).

Table 8. Comparison of general conditions between cases and controls

Category		Case group* (N=36) Freq. %		Control group (N=36) Freq. %		x^2	P
Educational level	<Middle school	27	75.0	23	63.9	1.05	>0.05
	Mid.scho & above	9	25.0	13	36.1		
Religious belief	Yes	5	13.9	4	5.6	2.85	>0.05
	No	31	84.1	68	94.4		
Belief about death**	Yes	11	30.6	12	33.3	0.06	>0.05
	No	25	69.4	24	66.7		

Note: * : Women who attempted suicide are referred to as the case group.
**: "Belief about death" means whether or not the interviewee believed in God and reincarnation.

2. Family structure

To understand the role of elders (mainly parents-in-law) in women's suicide, families were categorized into two types according to whether or not they lived with elders: nuclear families (small families) and linear families (large families). Nuclear families consist of a married couple, with or without unmarried children, while linear families consist of a married couple living with their parents.

Table 9 shows there was no significant difference in family structures between the suicide cases and the controls.

Table 9. Comparison of family structures between cases and controls

Family structure	Case group (N=36) Frequency	Case group (N=36) Percentage	Control group (N=36) Frequency	Control group (N=36) Percentage	x^2	P
Nuclear	15	41.7	14	38.9	0	>
Linear	21	58.3	22	61.1		

3. Relationship between husband and wife

It was found that the women who had attempted suicide were more likely to have quarreled with their husbands frequently. There were four women in the control group who had never quarreled with their husbands, while there was none in the case group (see Table 10).

Group	Often No.	Often %	Sometimes/Occasionally No.	Sometimes/Occasionally %	Never No.	Never %
Case (n=33)	9	27.3	24	72.7	0	0.0
Control (n=33)	1	3.0	28	84.9	4	12.1

4. Domestic violence and causes

It was also found that the women who had attempted suicide were more likely to have experienced domestic violence; 72.7% of the women who attempted suicide had been beaten by their husbands, compared with 33.3% of the women in the control group (see Table 11). The proportion "being beaten by husband in last year" among the women who had attempted suicide was 54.6%, significantly higher than that of the women in the control group (15.2%), which indicates that domestic violence is one of risk factors for rural women's suicide. The main reasons for domestic violence are family conflict (52.0%) and financial difficulties (32.0%).

Table 11. Comparison of domestic violence between cases and controls

Domestic violence		Case (n=33)		Control (n=33)		x^2	P
		No.	Percentage	No.	Percentage		
Beaten by husband	Yes	24	72.7	11	33.3	10.28	<0.05
	No	9	27.3	22	66.7		
Beaten by husband in last year	Yes	18	54.6	5	15.2	11.27	<0.05
	No	15	15.2	28	84.9		
Times beaten by husband	0	9	27.3	22	66.7	10.69	<0.05
	1-4	16	48.5	6	18.2		
	>5	8	24.2	5	15.2		
Reason for violence	Family conflict	13	52.0	2	16.2		
	Financial difficulty	8	32.0	7	63.6		
	Marital problems	3	12.0	1	9.1		
	Others	1	4.0	1	9.1		

It was learnt from focus group discussions with villagers that domestic violence is common in rural areas, with the husband usually beating the wife. Husbands beat their wives with fists and/or feet, while in severe cases a husband may hit his wife with sticks or farm tools.

In focus group discussions, villagers described "husbands beating wives" as normal behaviour in their local communities:

> *It (husband beats wife) is normal here.*

> *If the wife does something wrong, she should be punished by the husband. Few wives haven't been beaten by their husbands.*

> *(When a husband beats his wife) he uses anything at hand to beat his wife, such as a brick or a hoe. The wife would go to hospital if wounded.*

Due to the lagging economic development in rural areas, financial problems have become a major cause of family conflicts. When the family cannot afford fertilizer or a child's tuition, conflict arises between the wife and the husband: the wives often blame their husbands for their inability to make money, while husbands beat their wives to vent their anger. Therefore, many family conflicts finally turn into domestic violence.

Respondents gave the following reasons for domestic violence:

> *Usually due to the woman's faults, household chores or kids*

> *Couples always fight over the kid. For example, the wife protects the kid when the husband wants to discipline the child, as the result, the husband beats the wife.*

> *When the kid gets sick, the husband blames and beats the wife for not taking good care of the kid.*

> *Poverty! When the woman blames the man for his incapacity to earn money and compares him with others who are rich, the man gets angry and beats her.*

> *When the family can't afford the kid's schooling, the woman scolds her husband for it. The man feels disgraced and beats the wife.*

> *Some men have lovers outside the home. In this case, even if his wife has no faults, he will find an excuse to beat her.*

> *When the man spends all the money on gambling and is questioned by his wife, there will be a quarrel and battle.*

> *Some men look down upon women and never treat them well. Battles may occur any time, even when they are farming or talking.*

In the focus group discussions, most villagers (both men and women) said they considered it wrong for husbands to beat their wives, but most of them claimed that a man was justified in beating his wife if the woman did not respect her parents-in-law or was incorrigibly lazy and neglected household chores. Only a few of them insisted that men should never beat their wives and that couples should discuss matters instead of quarrelling and fighting.

The attitude of the community to the issue of domestic violence is evident from the following excerpts from interviewees' statements:

> *The woman should be disciplined. The man has the final word in everything.*
>
> *It's wrong to beat her when she does nothing wrong, but right when she makes mistakes.*
>
> *If the woman did something wrong and irritated the man, she should be punished with fists.*
>
> *If the wife lent something to others without getting the permission of her husband, she deserves the punishment of being beaten by the husband.*
>
> *Couples in rural areas, unlike people in the city, don't know how to communicate well. The woman deserves the beating when she does something wrong. If she doesn't obey her husband, or if she looks down upon her husband, she deserves the beating, also.*
>
> *Beating my wife is the only way to end the war between us. When I am annoyed by her, I beat her. That's the way to release my anger and to make her shut up. Then everything gets ok.*
>
> *It is wrong to beat a woman. Men and women are equal. They should discuss the issues with each other.*

Some women cannot bear domestic violence anymore and commit suicide after being beaten. It was found in individual in-depth interviews with women who had attempted suicide that many had been suffering from domestic violence before their suicide attempt. Doctors, when interviewed, also indicated that 30% to 40% of women admitted to hospital after attempting suicide had wounds and scars on their faces or limbs. Most of them were not serious, but 90% of the wounds were caused by their husbands.

One doctor described a case as follows:

> *Some women we rescued had fresh wounds. The injuries were not severe, just some bruises on the skin. Most were caused by their husbands' beatings. Usually these women are from families in poverty. It seems that financial problems are the main cause of family conflict.*

Another doctor said:

> *Around 30%-40% of reproductive-aged women rescued by us have wounds, more or less, but not severe, just on the face, arms or legs. I also remember that there was one woman with severe wounds all over her body. We were told that she was beaten by her husband with a rope. Most of the injures, i.e. about 90%, are from domestic violence. Women usually commit suicide by taking poison, no matter if rich or poor. This is the common characteristic of women's suicide.*

5. Family cohesion and adaptability

Sixty-nine women out of the 36 pairs of cases and controls participated in an investigation concerning family cohesion and adaptability (the fifth section of the questionnaire). The other three women did not take part because they had not lived with their families in the last month of the investigation period. To facilitate data analysis, those three women were given average scores. A paired t-test showed significant differences in family cohesion between the two groups. The control group had a higher level of family cohesion than the case group, which indicates that the women in the control group had closer emotional bonding among their family members than the women who had attempted suicide. There was no statistical difference between the two groups in terms of family adaptability (see Table 12).

Table 12. Comparison of family cohesion and adaptability between the two groups

Category	Case (n=36) Mean	95% CI	Control (n=36) Mean	95% CI	t*	P
Cohesion	55.33	(51.46, 59.20)	61.19	(58.10, 64.28)	2.04	<0.05
Adaptability	33.94	(30.92, 36.91)	37.74	(34.73, 40.76)	1.76	>0.05

*The scores for the two groups were normally distributed; therefore a paired t-test was used.

After analysing cases and controls, a cumulative frequency distribution of family cohesion showed 33.3% of them had a family cohesion score of less than 55, and 66.8% no higher than 63. Therefore, 55 and 63 were used as the dividing scores which classified family cohesion into three levels evenly, with one third of women in each level. Supposing the effect of family cohesion on suicide is the same in each level, a conditional logistic regression shows family cohesion as a protective factor for women's suicide (OR = 0.53, 95% CI: 0.25-0.99).

Table 13. Odds ratio of suicide – High family cohesion vs. low family cohesion

Family Cohesion	Case (n=36) No.	%	Control (n=36) No.	%	OR	95%CI	x^2	P
<55	14	38.9	7	19.4				
55-63	14	38.9	15	41.7	0.53	(0.25, 0.99)	3.86	<0.05
>63	8	22.2	14	38.9				

Family cohesion reflects emotional bonding among family members, including good communication, caring and helping each other. The women interviewed mentioned the importance of family cohesion:

Lo argued:

> If there had been somebody comforting me or consoling me at that time, I would not have taken the poison. But my husband just slept in another room, leaving me alone.

Luan said:

> I went mad from anger after quarrelling with my father-in-law. I thought when I lay in bed, that I would feel better when my husband came back at night and said warm words to me. I waited and waited, but he didn't come back. I took the poison the next morning.

6. Depression

All cases and controls were screened using the Beck Depression Inventory (BDI) to evaluate depression within one week of attempting suicide or being admitted to hospital. The average scores for cases was 17.86 and for controls 11.06. Thus there was a significant difference in the scores between the two groups, the case group having a higher depression score than the control group (see Table 14).

Table 14. Comparison of depression between cases and controls

	Case (n=36) Mean	95%CI	Control (n=36) Mean	95%CI	t*	P
Depression score	17.86	(13.93-21.80)	11.06	(8.69-13.42)	9.48	<0.01

*The scores for the two groups were normally distributed; therefore a paired t-test was used.

Based on their BDI scores, the cases and controls were categorized into two groups: without depression (normal or slight disturbance) and with depression (mild depression, moderate depression and severe depression). Of the women who had attempted suicide, 55.6% had experienced depressive symptoms within one week of their suicide attempts, compared with 30.6% in the control group. Thus the depression rates between cases and controls showed significant difference (see Table 15).

Table 15. Comparison of depression rates between cases and controls

Depression	Case (n=36) No.	%	Control (n=36) No.	%	χ^2	P
With depression	20	55.6	11	30.6	4.59	<0.05
Without depression	16	44.4	25	69.4		

Comparison of symptoms of depression between cases and controls indicated that the cases were more likely to have feelings of guilt, self-punishment and self-abhorrence, and suicidal intentions, than the controls (see Table 16). Here, "self-punishment" means that the interviewee felt herself being, or likely to be, punished; "self-abhorrence" describes a feeling of disgust, hate and disappointment with oneself; "feeling of guilt" refers to the interviewee feeling guilty and blaming herself; and "suicidal intention" means that the interviewee had suicidal ideas and would be likely to attempt suicide when triggered by certain events.

As shown in Tables 14, 15 and 16, women in the case group were more likely to experience depression within one week of attempting suicide. For women with symptoms of depression, the situation would be worsened when they were involved in conflict with family members and had poor communication, and not enough attention was paid to them within the family. The possibility of suicide attempts would increase markedly.

Table 16. Comparison of rates of depression symptoms between cases and controls

Symptoms	Cases (%)	Controls (%)	χ^2	P
Self-punishment	50.0	22.2	6.02	<0.05
Self-abhorrence	58.3	25.0	8.23	<0.05
Feeling of guilt	63.9	38.9	4.50	<0.05
Suicide intention	55.6	19.4	10.01	<0.05

7. Life events

As shown in Table 17, there was no significant difference in positive life events between the case and control groups; however, the score for negative life events was significantly higher in the case group (44.85) than in the control group (28.15). The negative life event score reflects mental distress: the higher the score, the more severe the impact on physical and psychological health from the negative event.

Table 17. Comparison of life event scores between case and control groups

Category	Cases (n=36)	Controls (n=36)	P
Positive life events	36.19	36.81	>0.05
Negative life events	44.85	28.15	<0.05

Analysis of each life event shows two events with a significant difference between the two groups: poor marital relationship and marital separation longer than one month. Two other events, financial difficulty and having a debt over Yuan 500 (US$ 62), were found to be significant at the level of $\alpha = 0.1$ (see Table 18).

Table 18. Univariate analysis of life events

Category		Cases (N=36) No.	Cases (N=36) Percentage	Controls (N=36) No.	Controls (N=36) Percentage	χ^2	P
Marital relationship	Good	28	77.8	35	97.2	6.22	<0.05
	Poor	8	22.2	1	2.8		
≥ 1month marital separation	Yes	4	11.1	0	0.0	--	<0.05*
	No	32	88.9	36	100.0		
Financial difficulty	Yes	16	44.4	9	25.0	3.00	<0.1
	No	20	55.6	27	75.0		
Having a debt over 500 Yuan	Yes	13	36.1	6	16.7	3.53	<0.1
	No	23	63.9	30	83.3		

* calculated from the Fisher exact probability test

After categorizing all 48 life event variables using cluster analysis, the significant variables in the univariate analysis were allocated into two clusters (see Table 19).

Table 19. Cluster analysis of life events

Category	Variable
Cluster 1	Poor marital relationship >1month Marital separation Unsatisfactory sexual life or singleness Husband' extramarital love affair
Cluster 2	Financial Difficulties Having a debt over 500 Yuan injury or illness of family members

Cluster 1 was related to the relationship between the couple, and Cluster 2 to economic variables. Therefore they were defined as 'marital factors' and 'financial factors'. The correlation coefficient between marital factors and financial factors was -0.06, indicating that marital status was unrelated to economic status; or, good marital relationship did not depend on good economic status.

8. Multivariate analysis

Univariate predictors with a p value < 0.05 (including 'beaten by husband'; 'beaten by husband in the last year'; 'feeling of guilt, self-punishment, self-abhorrence'; 'suicidal intention'; 'negative life events score'; 'family cohesion'; and 'conflict between the couple') were enrolled in a multivariate conditional logistic regression analysis.

As shown in Table 20, when statistical significance was defined as p ≥0.05, two variables, 'beaten by husband in last year' and 'suicidal intention', were risk factors for suicide. Another two variables 'beaten by husband' and 'negative life events' were significant risk factors for suicide at the level of 0.1.

Table 20. Results of multivariate conditional logistic regression analysis

Variable	OR	95% CL	χ^2	P
Beaten by husband	7.77	0.49, 123.64	2.11	<0.10
Beaten by husband in last year	97.79	1.30, 999	4.33	<0.05
Suicidal intention	39.16	1.97, 778	5.78	<0.05
Negative life events	3.50	0.85, 14.49	2.99	<0.10

Two factors, *f1* and *f2*, were identified through factor analysis of univariate predictors: *f1*, called the negative event factor, included the variables 'beaten by husband', 'beaten by husband in last year', 'negative life events', and 'conflict between the couple', all of which enhanced the chances of suicide attemps; *f2*, called the individual factor, represented the variables 'depression score' and 'family cohesion'. Depression scores were positively related to suicide (facilitating suicide), while family cohesion was negatively related to suicide (reducing suicide).

ATTITUDE TO SUICIDE

A questionnaire investigation was conducted with women in the control group to gain an understanding of their attitudes towards suicidal behaviour. It showed that most of them had a negative attitude. None blamed the family members involved, but they held different views - positive, neutral or negative - regarding the women who had committed or attempted suicide (see Table 21).

Table 21. Attitudes of women in control group to suicide

Category	Positive/ understanding*		Neutral		Negative/ opposing**	
	No.	%	No.	%	No.	%
To suicidal behaviour	0	0.0	13	36.1	23	63.9
To suicides	3	8.3	21	58.3	12	33.3
To suicide's family	11	30.6	25	69.4	0	0.0
To euthanasia	9	25.0	12	33.3	15	41.7

*: 'Positive/understanding' means holding a tolerant, accepting or approving attitude to suicide;
**: 'Negative/opposing' means discriminating against or objecting to suicide.

1. **Attitudes to suicidal behaviour**

    1.1 Negative attitude

    As shown in Table 21, most women in the control group held negative or opposing attitudes towards suicide. It was also learnt from interviewing villagers, public health officials and women who had attempted suicide, that most of them considered suicide as 'wrong behaviour'. They argued that suicide attempts hurt the person involved, but also had negative impacts on families and society. They said that suicide could not solve any problems but, on the contrary, it led the situation from bad to worse. There was always a solution to every problem, and suicide was not a good solution. The attitudes of interviewees toward suicidal behaviour are shown in the following excerpts:

    One public health official expressed frustration with people who give up too easily when the going gets rough:

    It is meaningless to die, and to be alive is always better than dead. Why? First, for the woman herself, she should have confidence in life. The difficulty is only temporary, and life will become better and better. No river can't be crossed; and no mountain can't be climbed. Just try the best that you can. Second, for the family and kids, their lives would be miserable without the wife and mother. Third, for society, her parents should be supported by her, and she can't give up the responsibility for the care of her parents. Finally, her suicide will also cause some negative impacts on the community and people living within it.

    Another public health official agreed:

    A woman's suicide is completely avoidable and unnecessary, because there is nothing serious. These small matters could happen at any time. The main problem is people don't change their irrational, negative thoughts into rational and positive thoughts. If we can help them channel their thoughts, it may not occur.

One member of the Women's Federation argued that:

It shouldn't happen. If the husband has an extramarital affair, she can leave him, or she can divorce him, can't she? She can live without him! If her husband beats her, she can also come here for help.

One hospital doctor agreed:

Women's suicide is a kind of abnormal phenomenon. Sometimes, we doctors tell them "you shouldn't commit suicide, it is silly. You have your parents to consider, for your kids sake too......".

1.2 Positive attitude

Although most of interviewees thought that women should not commit suicide, some still considered it was justified in certain situations, such as when the woman had done something 'immoral' or faced a difficulty that could not be settled. They considered suicide an alternative way to solve problems.

The following excerpts from individual in-depth interviews illustrate this more accepting attitude to suicide. Surprisingly, two of the sources of this attitude were health authorities (charged with the responsibility for defending health and longevity in populations) and doctors (bound by the Hippocratic Oath at an individual level).

One Health Bureau official defended suicide in some situations:

A woman has the right to commit suicide when facing the following situations: when she feels life is hopeless and meaningless, she could commit suicide, or when she cannot escape from her bitter living environment. For example, one woman got married to a Muslim. One of the family members had a dream saying that the woman was a curse, a bane, then the family member began to abuse her. In that situation, nobody could save her. Besides, if the woman did something immoral, such as elopement or adultery etc., she could commit suicide; or if she were terminally ill and suffering, she could choose euthanasia.

One hospital doctor also provided a qualified defence of suicide:

She indeed had no other choice. Considering the bad relationship with her husband, and conflict with her mother-in-law etc., even we thought that she should commit suicide.

One villager also suggested that, in some circumstances, self-inflicted death may be preferable to a miserable life, or financial concerns may justify suicide:

Sometimes it (suicide) is the best way to solve problems. Deep poverty, painful disease, and hard life, maybe death is better.

If I had a severe disease, the family could not afford the treatment. So the only way would be suicide.

1.3 Neutral attitude

In the control group, 36.1% of the women held neutral attitudes toward suicide (see Table 21). Some villagers also had an ambiguous attitude to suicidal behaviour, and had no further comments on women's suicide. As they said,

I have nothing to say. Suicide is common here, it's not special.

Sometimes, rural women just intend to threaten others by committing suicide. It is nothing serious. I have no idea about it.

Thus there is a degree of normalization of suicide as an inevitable solution to a variety of problems.

2. Attitudes towards suicide victims and their families

Most of interviewees had sympathy for suicide victims and the families involved. They said they would like to keep up interaction with those women who had attempted suicide and their families, and even be more friendly towards them.

They suggested the following forms of support:

> *We will give a hand to them whenever they face difficulties, and I will keep friendship with them as before, such as cooking for their kids.*

> *It is an unfortunate thing for all families. We are living in the same village. Of course we will help them. Who knows the future? Maybe someday my family will also face such a thing. We should help each other.*

> *Previously we didn't have a close relationship with them, but now we should have more concern for them since they have encountered this unlucky thing. I believe they would appreciate any help at the moment.*

3. Impact of suicide

The interviewees all agreed that suicides have negative impacts on individuals, families and society, especially on families. It is hard for families to cope with the aftermath of a suicide.

The following represents interviewees' opinions on the impact of suicide, covering the financial, societal and emotional costs of a women's premature death:

One public health official took a macro perspective on the impact of suicide:

> *A woman's suicide has a negative impact on society. Most people consider it shameful to commit suicide. For her family, it is a sudden and unexpected shattering of their lives. The family may never get out of the shadow. Maybe the family had been in debt for the wedding. Now the woman has died and more money will be spent on the funeral. The family will become poorer and probably never have a good life again. In addition, it also brings deep grief and sorrow to the children whose mother has committed suicide. This traumatic experience can cause serious life-long damage to the children. They will be more likely to have problems in their studies and future lives.*

Similarly, one member of the Women's Federation emphasized the societal impact:

> *First, women's suicides make the society unstable and produce some negative impacts. It harms the stability of the society. For the family, the mother's suicide has an irrevocable impact on the child's mind.*

One doctor suggested suicide was a symptom of societal problems:

> *It brings extra burdens to society, the family and people involved. For families, the influence is tremendous and hard to measure, especially for the kids, this is an incurably traumatic experience. It also causes grief and loss to her parents and relatives. The increase in suicides reveals some social problems as well.*

While one of the villagers emphasized the effects on the family:

> *Of course it will have some bad influences. When the wife dies, the husband can't live well under the huge pressure, both economic and emotional pressure. The family will break down. On the contrary, the influence on society is less severe.*

> *It will bring some inconvenience. If the wife dies, no one does the housework, no one does the cooking; if the husband dies, no one earns money.*
>
> *Others have a wife, and he has none; other children have a mother, while his have none.*
>
> *It brings tremendous stress to the family. Without a wife, the man has nobody to talk with and be company for him at home. Without a mother, the kids lack care and will become problematic in the future.*

4. Attitudes of women who had attempted suicide

Most of the women who had attempted suicide realized that their suicidal behaviour had caused a negative impact on their families and children, and said that they would not attempt suicide in future, even if they encountered similar problems and difficulties. However, several women hesitated and did not exclude the possibility of committing suicide in the future.

SUICIDE PREVENTION

There are no specific institutions or organizations devoted to suicide prevention in Longde County, except for the Women's Federation, which aims to protect women's rights and help them to solve their problems. However, their services are tragically underutilized because many women have never heard of the Federation.

According to local health officials and the Women' Federation, there are some problems and obstacles in suicide prevention. First, the local government has not paid enough attention to suicide and has made little effort to address the problem; cooperation and collaboration across governmental departments is severely lacking, and there is no department committed to suicide prevention. Second, insufficient funding, personnel training and equipment have been allocated to the prevention of suicide. In addition, it is hard to improve education and change traditional ideas in rural areas within a short period of time. Local people do not realize the severity of the problem. It is important, but difficult to teach them how to prevent suicidal behaviour. Third, in some quarters, including parts of the health sector, suicide and suicide attempts are the norm and, in some cases, interviewees provided qualified justification for suicide attempts.

Although people have different ideas on how to prevent suicide, they have some thoughts in common, including mobilizing society and increasing awareness of the problem; changing traditional ideas; improving women's social position; and strengthening management and regulation of mouse-poison sales and storage. The following suggestions for a comprehensive strategy to prevent suicidal behaviour were selected from the interviews with local health workers:

> One of public health officials emphasized education:
>
> > *First, self-protection is important for women. We should develop and disseminate educational messages on prevention of suicide. People haven't realized it in the past, but if we pay enough attention to it now, people will be aware of this problem. We could use some vivid examples to tell people why it happens, and how to deal with it. For instance, people can choose divorce as a way and use the law to resolve conflicts. People should realize that life is the primary right of every individual. Without it, other things become nonsense. However, many rural women do not seem to realize that.*
>
> > *The second thing is to reinforce the management of mouse poison and the third is to increase public awareness of the law. Some matters are unable to be settled within families, so we should let women be aware that they can choose a formal way to cope with their troubles. According to previous experiences, some matters may be mediated by the village commission or resident committee. Currently, although a husband beating a wife does not seem common, domestic violence still exists. Thus we should reinforce education on the equality of men and women. By doing that, we could decrease violent behaviour and prevent suicide caused by domestic violence.*

Domestic violence emerged as a key explanatory factor in many of the interviews, but in one case, a public health official argued that it was decreasing in prevalence.

Domestic violence exists in some families, about 10%-20% of families. Compared with before, it has become much better now. This is a kind of social improvement. I grew up in a rural area, and I felt domestic violence in the past was much more severe than now in rural areas. As I know, some women commit suicide because of domestic violence. Some of them had been tortured by their husbands for a long time.

Prevention strategies proposed by public officials emphasized legal changes and training and health education for front-line officials and health care providers, as well as cross-sectoral cooperation.

If I were asked to provide a feasible proposal to prevent women from suicide, I would emphasize increasing awareness of the law and improving government participation. The government should support it, and pay more attention to it. Collaboration across governments, judicial departments and the Women's Federation is effective in promoting education. Women will be taught how to protect themselves.

Regular channels should be established through which some family problems can be resolved. At village level, the village commission should take the responsibility for mediating family conflict. When a case occurs, they can resolve it, or let someone who has received relevant training explain the situation to the woman. If some issue needs to be resolved by law, it should come to court. If Women's Federation help is needed, they should come to the Federation. If the woman still experiences mental distress, they should give her valuable suggestions to help her release the pressure.

Furthermore, hospital involvement in suicide prevention is crucial. Physicians should improve their abilities in emergency and routine treatment. Health education, especially in the media, is very important, too. To sum up, the village commission plays the critical role in the whole process.

One doctor's proposal involved improving women's status in the family, in law and in society as a whole:

One strategy is to elevate women's position in the family; another is to increase women's knowledge about the law and their awareness of self-salvation. The truth is that it is very difficult to improve women's family position. If a woman has certain economic power, and her economic position increases, her family position will improve correspondingly. Isn't that right? The problem is that the majority of rural women don't earn money. They are financially dependent on their husbands. If they were independent, the violence would decrease.

To increase women's awareness about the law, we could train them in the village or township. This is one side. The other side is to raise the law awareness of the kids through education at primary school or secondary school. Then the kids could give their mothers some suggestions when the mothers face difficulties.

Villagers had a variety of suggestions, including:

Men and women should understand each other, earning money by hand, share the work, and no gossip.

Men work outside, and women work at home looking after the kids. Men should understand the woman's hard work in taking care of kids and family.

If the woman's social position was elevated, and the traditional idea that the man is superior and the woman inferior changed, family conflict would decrease, men wouldn't beat women, and women wouldn't commit suicide.

The neighbours could mediate family conflict. Besides, education is necessary. Since women are lacking knowledge, women's classes should aim at the family and teaching them how to live.

Public awareness of the law should be increased. People should be taught that suicide is not the right way to solve problems.

Thus there seems to be considerable overlap between the stakeholders in their suggestions for prevention strategies. The suggestions include regulating the sale of mouse poison, legal reform, health sector reform, economic reforms to equalize access to resources, improved formal and informal education about gender relations, and training of officials and workers to identify problem signs at the local level and to refer appropriately. However, one important challenge remains for those charged with preventing suicide. The normalization of both suicide and domestic violence, which the interviews revealed, is a major obstacle to change. To argue that both suicide and domestic violence are justified in some circumstances is contrary to basic human rights conventions and to the Hippocratic Oath taken by health professionals.

CHAPTER 5.
DISCUSSION AND SUGGESTIONS

DISCUSSION

1. Suicide methods

Among the 36 women who attempted suicide during the period of the study, 97.2% of them used poison. Thus, easy access to poisons and sleeping pills may be an important factor. It was learnt that, although illegal sales of lethal mouse poison have been forbidden by the local government, it can still be procured at local markets, making it easy for villagers to buy it. In addition, in most rural families, leftover pesticides are stored in the home. Easy access to these lethal materials is a major contributing factor for those who have severe conflict with their families or neighbours and commit suicide on impulse.

2. Reducing access to lethal means as an effective strategy to prevent suicide

Analysis of local data showed that, in previous years, about 100 women of child-bearing age women committed suicide every year. However, in the year under investigation, there was a sharp reduction to only 41 suicides in the county. It was learnt from interviewing local people that, in previous years, mouse poison was easily available and could be found in the home. However, from late 2001 to 2002, the local Patriotic Sanitation Campaign Commission and the Police Department launched a campaign to eliminate illegal sales of lethal mouse poison. When access to the means of self-harm was restricted, the number of suicides by self-poisoning dropped. Therefore, limiting access to lethal means of suicide is one effective way to prevent suicide attempts.

3. Motivation for suicide

Three types of motivation were identified for rural women's suicides: on impulse, to escape from difficulties, and to threaten others.

Women who attempt suicide to escape from difficulties display the most individualized psychological state. Their pessimism escalates progressively over a period, developing from dissatisfaction with something into final world-weariness. They usually do not attempt suicide on impulse; instead they contemplate it for some time before taking action. This was the only type of suicide in the study that demonstrated self-control and rational thought on behalf of the women, rather than impulse. From the perspective of psychiatry, most suicide victims of this type are prone to depression, which is also confirmed in this study: depression in the case group was found to be statistically higher than in the control group.

Women who attempt suicide on impulse make impetuous decisions and act under the influence of key events, but they usually regret it right away. Some women in the study had attempted suicide in temporary despair or anger after being scolded or beaten by their husbands, although they had enjoyed a good relationship previously.

The third type, who attempt suicide to threaten others, demonstrate behaviour with an interpersonal motivation, to control others or to achieve a goal. By displaying extreme behaviour, their intention is to gain sympathy, to arouse panic or to impose pressures on others. However, once they understand that their demands or desires cannot be met, they are most likely to turn the pretend suicide into a real suicidal act. In the study, it was found that some women had attempted suicide in order to push their husbands to give up domestic violence.

4. Causes of suicide

According to the study, family conflict is the leading cause of women's suicides. Lack of harmony between daughter-in-law and mother-in-low, conflict between the couple, and domestic violence are direct causes of suicide attempts. However, underlying those proximate causes are distal factors such as poverty, traditional customs, family environment, interpersonal relationships, the normalization of suicide and psychological factors.

4.1 Poverty

Poverty caused by lagging economic development is the major reason for family conflict. When money is short or needed urgently, a 'war' is triggered between the couple, tensions increase in the family and it is difficult to remain composed. Quarrels then develop into domestic violence. Women, who are more likely to be victims of domestic violence, might attempt suicide after quarrelling with or being beaten by their husbands. Therefore, poverty is an important triggering factor for women's suicides.

4.2 Traditional prejudices against women

Feudal beliefs, such as 'Man is superior to woman', and 'Carrying on the family line is the first task for women', and practices such as marriages arranged by parents, persist in rural areas. Therefore, the husband is believed to be superior and the wife inferior, and it is common for husbands to beat their wives. Arranged marriages and trade marriages are not rare in rural areas. Some families, in order to prepare for their son's marriage, ask for a high bride-price. Therefore the marriages are not based on love, but on material well-being and economic status and, as a result, it is hard for the couple to develop a happy, long-lasting relationship. Such feudal traditions make it more likely for women to become the victims of domestic violence.

4.3 Family environment

A large number of male adults from rural parts of Longde County migrate into cities for work, leaving the women at home to take on the dual responsibilities of home and work. The women, not only engage in housework such as caring for children, cooking, washing and cleaning, but are also responsible for farm work in their husbands' absence. Thus rural women suffer from poverty and burdensome work, which makes them particularly vulnerable to mental distress and suicide attempts.

4.4 Psychological factors

Poor living conditions, a huge struggle just to survive, and lack of access to quality culture and education, has thrown rural women into a spiritual 'desert'. Such closed environments produce an unhealthy psychological state and have considerable impact on women's personalities. As the collective economy declines, interpersonal relationships are becoming more distant, and this is being further exacerbated by a lack of any social support system. As a consequence, women do not receive enough social support and help when facing a variety of difficulties.

The study illustrated significant differences between the case and control groups in the mental distress they felt one week before their suicide attempts. The cases experienced sadness, unhappiness and self-blame, and already had suicidal tendencies. They would be likely to attempt suicide when stimulated by an appropriate trigger.

4.5 Normalization of suicide

The interviews revealed a degree of justification for suicide based on economic, moral or health grounds. Although only a few interviewees actively supported suicide under some circumstances, over 36% of the women in the control group and a number of official interviewees held neutral attitudes to suicide. Thus there is a degree of normalization of suicide and suicide attempts, which presents a challenge to suicide prevention programmes. The same challenge is present for those concerned about preventing domestic violence, one of the key causes of suicide attempts.

5. Reasons for domestic violence

Domestic violence is an important cause of suicide among women. There are several main reasons for domestic violence:

5.1 Historical reasons

The feudal belief in the 'authority of the husband' and 'the woman's subordinate role' has been deeply rooted in rural areas of China for thousands of years. Discrimination against women remains a serious social problem, manifesting itself in several forms. First, violence against women is considered normal and is validated by custom. Second, carrying on the ancestral line is regarded as the first priority of women, and a woman's inability to have a son for her husband can lead to family violence. Some husbands do not welcome the birth of daughters, and beat and abuse their wives if they do not bear sons. In some cases, a man may force his wife to divorce him, thus allowing him to re-marry and re-procreate. Third, Longde society does not take domestic violence seriously and regards it as an individual or household affair. When the victims of such violence come to the village committee or the Women's Federation for help, these organizations, at most, mediate between the couple, rather than making use of the law to defend the victims' rights and educating the couples about the law and their rights.

5.2 Individual factors

The intrinsic reason for domestic violence, for both victims and offenders, is that their overall quality of life is relatively low. The offenders, who do not have knowledge of the law and 'morality', think that violence against women is the normal course of events to discipline an erring wife. On the other hand, the victims, who are usually poorly educated and not informed about the law and women's rights, are obedient towards their husbands and endure the abuse silently.

5.3 Social factors

The greater mobility of the male labour force in Longde County over the past decade has had significant effects on the social fabric in rural areas. First, men's absence from their villages for long periods to work in the cities has compromised the traditional value of marital fidelity. This, along with the emerging ethos of sexual liberation, may have triggered an increase in the incidence and/or awareness of extramarital affairs in rural areas. This in turn appears to be one of the contributing factors in domestic violence. Although no such case was identified in this study and some public officials argued that domestic violence is actually declining, local members of the Women's Federation reported that extramarital affairs had caused a rapid rise in family violence and the break-up of marriages.

Second, current research suggests that changing patterns in the sexual division of labour, necessitated by men's long periods of absence working in cities, have contributed to an increased incidence of suicide attempts amongst women left with the burden of total responsibility for domestic and farm work.

5.4 Law and regulations

An important reason for the high prevalence of domestic violence is a lack of a sound and wholesome system of justice in the area of family violence. Even where such laws are in place, they are rarely implemented. First, violence against women usually happens in the home; the victims are not willing to expose the family 'skeletons', while the neighbors do not want to intrude in the private lives of others, hence it remains hidden and ignored. Second, it is hard to bring the relevant laws, such as the Constitution, Criminal Law, Marriage Law, Law on Women's Rights, Law on Public Security, to bear because of their abstract nature. As a result, when sanctions are suggested or implied by some organizations, they are not commensurate with the seriousness and consequences of the acts because the cases are considered family disputes rather than criminal acts. Since women are not protected effectively by the law, domestic violence against women is rampant.

6. Reasons for women's suicides

A variety of reasons for women's suicide were proposed in this study based on the information from the questionnaire investigation with those women who had attempted suicide and the controls, in-depth interviews with informants and focus group discussions.

As shown in Figure 2 below, women living in poor and closed environments work hard at domestic chores and farming all of their lives and suffer from low status in society and violence within the family. Lacking available legal mechanisms and social support systems, women are more inclined to become helpless and depressed when being abused and might therefore choose suicide as a way to resolve their difficulties and relieve their intense sadness. To sum up, women's suicide is the result of the interaction between societal, environmental, family and individual factors. Poverty is often the source of conflict and a degree of societal normalization of suicide (as a justifiable solution to difficulties) forms the backdrop for solutions to that conflict. Family conflict and the accompanying domestic violence are triggering factors, and easy access to lethal poisons is the facilitating factor for suicide attempts.

Figure 2. Factors in women's suicide attempts

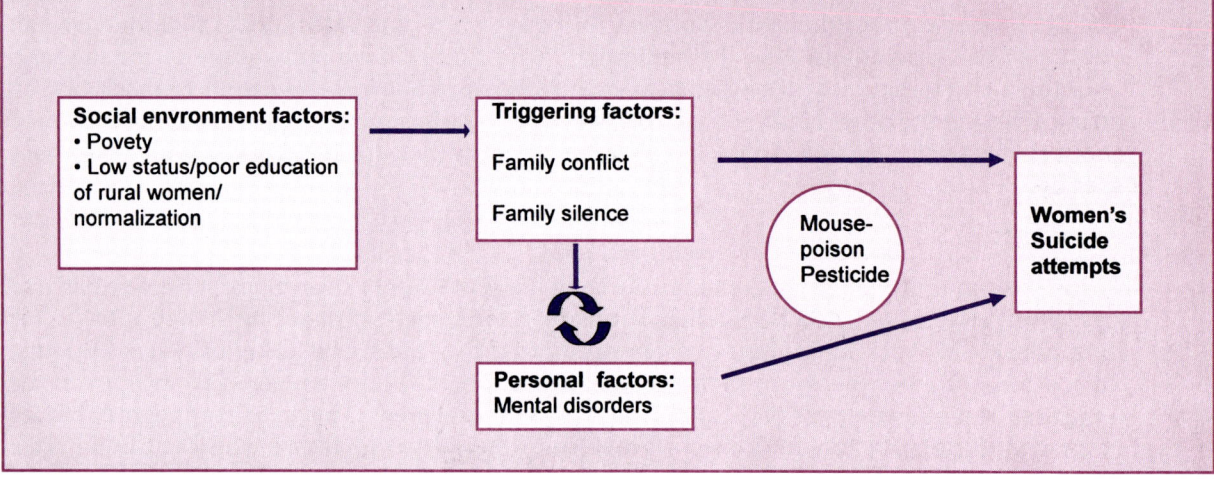

SUGGESTIONS FOR PREVENTION

1. Restrict access to means of suicide

In comparing data from this study with previous statistics, it was found that the number of suicides dropped sharply after the government started controlling sales of lethal mouse poisons. Therefore, removing potentially lethal materials from the environment and restricting access to the means of suicide is one of the most effective measures to prevent suicide.

Measures that reduce access to lethal means of suicide could include:

- improving cooperation between local health departments and other governmental departments on management of mouse poison, and restricting any illegal sale or distribution of lethal mouse poisons;
- establishing regulations on pesticide management, and assigning pest management personnel to manage, store and dispense the pesticide; and
- developing new mouse poisons and pesticides of low toxicity and high effect.

2. Improve rural women's quality of life

There is a need for local rural organizations to develop public education campaigns on cherishing life, to educate people on the severity and cost of suicide to the individual, the family and society, and to inform people that suicide cannot solve any problem. People can learn better ways to deal with their difficulties.

Special training sessions are needed for rural women to improve communication skills in their families. The study found that rural women had attempted suicide mostly after quarrelling with their husbands; most women had scolded their husbands with hurtful words that had injured the husband's self-esteem and had resulted in domestic violence. Accordingly, it is necessary to enhance women's and men's communication skills in the family, teaching them how to communicate with others, how to build up good relationships as couples, and how to handle their problems calmly.

Psychological services should be made available to the public. Specific psychological consultations and treatment should be conducted among those populations identified as being at high risk for suicide attempts, improving their ability to adapt to society and deal with crises, and teaching them to value their lives. Suicide prevention programmes and organizations should mobilize relatives, friends, neighbours, colleagues and community workers to address victims' specific problems, provide sufficient support and comfort to them, and keep in close contact with them. Such measures could effectively eliminate their loneliness and despair, enhance their attachment to their families and also increase their confidence.

3. Improve women's position in the family and society

Interventions should be carried out to transform social traditions and eliminate the feudal belief that men are superior to women, as well as harmful practices such as arranged marriages and trade marriages. The belief that women should enjoy equal rights with men in all spheres of life should be advocated, including that women should have equal rights to choose love and marriage freely, and that women have equal rights and responsibilities for their own lives.

Society should recognize and affirm the significance and value of women's work and, through this, increase women's dignity and love of life, helping them to build up positive and healthy values and attitudes.

A joint effort should also be made to improve the local economy and create employment opportunities for women and, by so doing, to increase family income and reduce conflict between husbands and wives.

4. Eliminate and prevent domestic violence

Moral and legal education should be enforced to improve people's quality of life, their access to informed decision-making and their understanding of the law. To raise general awareness of the hazards of domestic violence and guide people to regulate their family relationships within the law, contract issues could be explained in a user-friendly way by illustrating with case analyses.

To achieve success in preventing domestic violence, collaboration across a broad spectrum of agencies must be fostered to ensure that prevention efforts are comprehensive and to expedite legislation on preventing such violence. An integrated judicial system is the key to preventing and eliminating domestic violence. So far, domestic violence against women is tolerated publicly and is not recognized by society as a crime. Violence, as defined by law, ranges from abuse or mild injury to serious injury or death. However, domestic violence is not listed or defined clearly in existing laws. Due to its abstract nature, it is hard to pass judgement on domestic violence against women. Only when domestic violence becomes a severe crime will it be considered a criminal act.

It is imperative that domestic violence be considered a problem rather than the norm. Major media campaigns, covering print, audio and visual media, could bombard the population with messages about what constitutes domestic violence and violence against women, and that it is not acceptable anywhere in the world under any circumstances. Such campaigns have been tried with a considerable degree of success in other countries.

Shelters should be established to offer protection to the victims of domestic violence, where they can receive treatment for physical and psychological wounds and also be taught about the law and empowerment.

5. Pay particular attention to attempted suicide

After being rescued, persons who have attempted suicide usually become excessively sensitive to their surroundings and others people's attitudes, and they fear prejudice and discrimination from many quarters. Therefore, the attitude of others is crucial in treatment and intervention for those who have attempted suicide. People (especially health professionals rescuing the suicide attempters) should be affirming, composed and confident in treatment and support.

Those in contact with a woman who has attempted suicide should not make moral judgements on suicidal behaviour and the philosophy behind suicide during the crucial period immediately after the suicide attempt. Temporary hospitalization at this stage may prove an effective short-term protective measure. Such a neutral environment may facilitate amelioration of instigating circumstances in the family environment and be a suitable venue for the assessment of mental status and risk of future suicide attempts. Psychological consultation and treatment should be offered to suicide attempters at the hospital.

6. Establish suicide prevention centres and implement integrated prevention programmes

Effective suicide prevention programmes should be developed and implemented, for instance, by establishing a Life-hotline (suicide hotline), providing access to psychological consultation, and building up suicide prevention centres. In addition, health education should be conducted for the public. The whole society, especially families, schools and communities, should collaborate in promoting suicide prevention and changing the evasive and discriminatory attitudes towards suicide. Often a saturation media campaign using all media sources is the best way to start societal debate about issues such as suicide and domestic violence. Media messages emphasizing universal rights issues and identifying which attitudes and behaviours are negotiable, and which are not, seem to be most successful in changing societal norms.

Special attention should be paid to persons with suicidal tendencies, especially those expressing suicidal ideas or plans such as writing a posthumous letter or attempting suicidal acts. Recognizing the signs of suicide is significant in predicting subsequent suicidal behaviour. Therefore, persons with suicidal signs should be observed closely and particular attention paid to them.

REMAINING CHALLENGES

One of the most difficult challenges in suicide prevention is societal change, especially altering a pervasive approach to suicide (and domestic violence) which sees it as normal, to an approach which regards it as a problem, couched within human rights conventions. Those charged with such a task must adopt an intersectoral approach, collaborating with international agencies, national and local governmental and nongovernmental organizations, health authorities and providers, the media, educational institutions, the judiciary and law enforcement agencies, private enterprise, donor agencies and individuals in their local environments to develop programmes that are effective, affordable, accessible and, most importantly, acceptable, sensitive and user-friendly to consumers and providers. Examples of best practice from around the world can be made available to national and local policy-makers, service providers and consumers for consideration and adaptation to local requirements.

Suicide prevention does not stand alone as a public health challenge. As many of the interviewees in this study so eloquently put it, suicide (like domestic violence) is a mirror of social disquiet. Why do men feel so badly about themselves that they beat up their wives? Why do women and men feel so disempowered and desperate that self-inflicted harm and/or death appears to be the only solution to their problems? These are the basic questions about quality of life and social capital that a prevention programme needs to address, in conjunction with programmes on issues such as drug buse, depression, violence generally and disintegration of the sense of community

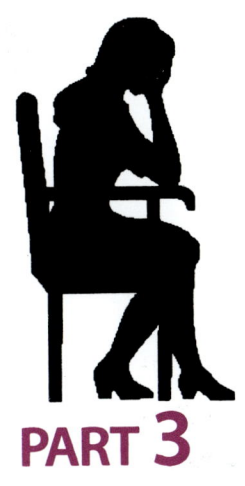

PART 3

Domestic violence against Pregnant Women and Its Impact : A Survey in Northern China

TABLE OF CONTENTS

Chapter 1. Introduction 58

    Domestic violence against women: global and regional situation 58

    Domestic violence against women in China 59

    Study objectives 60

Chapter 2. Literature review 61

    Characteristics of domestic violence against pregnant women 61

    Health consequences of domestic violence against pregnant women 63

    Domestic violence screening and intervention 64

    Conclusions 64

Chapter 3. Methodology 65

    Research design 65

    Research sites and time period 65

    Research methods 65

    Research instruments 66

    Training of interviewers 67

    Operational definitions 67

    Data processing and analysis 68

    Ethical considerations 68

Chapter 4. Domestic violence against women before, during and after pregnancy 68

    Results 69

        Women's characteristics 69

        Domestic violence situation 72

        Factors associated with domestic violence 76

        Effects of abuse on women's reproductive health 82

        Results of in-depth interviews with abused women 83

   Conclusions 89
    Prevalence of domestic violence 89
    Pattern of domestic violence 90
    Women's actions in response to domesticviolence 90
    Women's attitudes towards domestic violence 91
    and gender roles
    Possible factors associated with domestic violence 91
    Effects of domestic violence on reproductive health 93

Chapter 5. Domestic violence against women seeking abortions 93
   Results 93
    Respondents' characteristics 93
    Domestic violence among women seeking abortions .. 96
    Factors related to domestic violence 99
   Conclusions 104
    Domestic violence among women seeking abortions 104
    Sexual violence within the family 104
    Potential risk factors related to domestic violence 105

Chapter 6. Men's accounts of domestic violence 105
   Results 106
   Conclusions 109

Chapter 7. Maternal and child health workers' knowledge, attitudes 109
   and practices regarding domestic violence
   Results 110
   Conclusions 110

Chapter 8. Recommendations 111

Chapter 1.

INTRODUCTION

DOMESTIC VIOLENCE AGAINST WOMEN: GLOBAL AND REGIONAL SITUATION

Violence against women, including pregnant women, is a major public health issue both globally[1,2] and in the Western Pacific Region[3]. The World Report on Violence and Health reviewed 48 population-based surveys of intimate partner violence from across the globe (1982-1999) and found that "between 10% and 69% of women reported being physically assaulted by an intimate male partner at some point in their lives"[4]. The more recent WHO Multi-country Study on Women's Health and Domestic Violence against Women[4] found similar prevalence levels, with the lifetime prevalence of physical violence against women, by an intimate partner, varying from 13% to 61% across the ten countries studied. For sexual violence, the range was 6% to 59% and the range of lifetime prevalence of physical or sexual violence or both by an intimate partner was between 15% and 71%'[6]

Violence against women is not a new phenomenon. In the late 1970s, it was estimated that close to 4 million American women were being physically abused each year[7], and a study conducted in an American urban emergency department in the early 1980s found that 24% of women seen for any reason had a history of domestic violence[8]. Those figures significantly underrepresent the real levels of intimate partner violence, given that the taboos and shame associated with physical and psychological violence in the home contribute to serious underreporting[9]

A 1998 overview of prevalence rates in the Western Pacific Region found lifetime rates of violence against women varied between 22.5% (in an Australian study), 39% (in a Malaysian study by ARROW) and 61% (married women assaulted by their husbands in a South Korean study). Again, these figures are likely to represent the tip of the domestic violence iceberg, and do not report on the levels of psychological abuse.[10]

To understand the sources of the problem, and to develop appropriate prevention strategies, many disciplines must be involved in research and programme development, including those from both the health sciences and the social sciences. While violence against women generally, and pregnant women in particular, has severe health consequences, it is a social problem that warrants an immediate coordinated response from multiple sectors. The Declaration on the Elimination of Violence Against Women defines violence against women as "any act of gender-based violence that results in, or is likely to result in, physical, sexual or mental harm or suffering to women, including threats of such acts, coercion or arbitrary deprivation of liberty, whether occurring in public or in private life"[11].

---

[1] *World report on violence and health*. Geneva, World Health Organization, 2002.
[2] *WHO Multi-country Study on Women's Health and Domestic Violence against Women*. Geneva, World Health Organization, 2005.
[3] *Domestic violence: A priority public health issue in the Western Pacific Region*. Manila, World Health Organization, Western Pacific Regional Office, 1998.
[4] *Op cit.* Ref 1:89.
[5] *Op cit.* Ref 2.
[6] *Op cit.* Ref 2: 27.
[7] Straus MA, Gelles RJ, Steinmetz SK. Behind closed doors: violence in the American family. New York, Doubleday/Anchor, 1980.
[8] Goldberg WG, Tomlanovich MC. Domestic violence victims in the emergency department: New findings. *Journal of the American Medical Association*. 1984, 254: 3259-3264.
[9] *Op cit.* Ref 2.
[10] *Op cit.* Ref 3.
[11] United Nations, 1993.

Domestic violence against women is an underreported crime associated with serious health, social and economic consequences[12,13,14]. Domestic violence during pregnancy has been recognized as a major risk to the health of both the mother and the fetus or infant.[15] Previous studies have documented rates of abuse during pregnancy of from 5.5% to 17%, depending on the population studied and the screening method used, and that the problem may be largely unreported to health care providers[16,17,18]. The most recent comprehensive multicountry study on violence against women[19] shows that, although the reported rates of violence against pregnant women were less overall than those against all women in most sites, the rates were between 4% and 12%, which is alarming given the vulnerable situation of both the mother and her unborn child. Research indicates that violence during pregnancy may be a more prevalent problem than pregnancy-induced hypertension, gestational diabetes, or placenta previa, conditions for which pregnant women are routinely screened. Obstetrical manifestations of abuse include miscarriages, spontaneous abortion, low birth-weight, multiple abortions, placental separation, rupture of the uterus and preterm labour[20]. The short- and long-term psychological, emotional and social impacts on women, children, families and society as a whole are immeasurable.

Sexual coercion in any abusive relationship context places women at risk for all of the consequences of unprotected sex: unplanned pregnancy, HIV infection and other sexually transmitted diseases. Battered women, particularly when they are being sexually abused, may also experience dyspareunia and frequent vaginal and urinary tract infection[21]. Some studies have found that the prevalence of self-reported abuse in the population of women in early pregnancy who seek early pregnancy termination services is 31%-39.5%, and women in abusive relationships are more likely to consider termination[22,23]. Battered women are more likely to have been pregnant or to have miscarried or had an unwanted pregnancy than non-battered women.

Another study found that battering during pregnancy is associated with an increased severity and frequency of abuse, as well as an increased risk of depression, anxiety disorders, substance abuse and homicide[24]. Injury and death are only the most immediate, visible consequences of domestic violence. There is also some evidence that being battered is a significant risk factor for low-birth-weight babies and the maternal complication of low weight gain, as well as infection, anaemia, smoking and alcohol or drug abuse.

Thus past and recent epidemiological studies worldwide, and in the Western Pacific Region, indicate that domestic violence, including violence against pregnant women, is a major burden of disease, as well as a major public health, social and economic issue that remains largely underexplored.

DOMESTIC VIOLENCE AGAINST WOMEN IN CHINA

China was not included in the 2005 WHO Multi-country Study, but a systematic study of domestic violence, especially in rural parts of the country, is seriously overdue. It is difficult to obtain an accurate estimate of the frequency of domestic violence incidents in the country because of the persistence of

---

[12] Mahon L. Common characteristics of abused women. *Mental Health Nurse*. 1981, 3:137-157.
[13] Parikh, R. Violence meets its match. *Canadian Nurse*, October 1991: 14-15.
[14] Raiker, A. *Pregnancy, birthing and family planning in Kenya: changing patterns of behavior: a health utilization study in Kissei District*. Copenhagen, Center for Development Research, 1991.
[15] *The battered woman*. Washington, DC, American College of Obstetricians and Gynecologists, 1989 (Technical bulletin No. 124).
[16] McFarlane J et al. Assessing for abuse during pregnancy: Severity and frequency of injuries and associated entry into prenatal care. *Journal of the American Medical Association*, 1992, 267:3176-8.
[17] Hillard PJ. Physical abuse in pregnancy. *Obstetrics and Gynecology*, 1985, 66:185-90.
[18] Berenson A et al. Drug abuse and other risk factors for physical abuse in pregnancy among white non-Hispanic, black, and Hispanic women. *American Journal of Obstetrics and Gynecology*, 1991, 164:491-9.
[19] *Op cit*. Ref 2.
[20] Parker B, McFarlane J, Soeken K. Abuse during pregnancy: Effects on maternal complications and birth weight in adult and teenage women. *Obstetrics and Gynecology*, 1994, 84:323-8.
[21] Carole W. Identification, assessment and intervention with victims of domestic violence. In: Warshaw, C, Ganley A. eds. Improving the health care response to violence: a resource manual for health care providers. Family Violence Prevention Fund, 1998
[22] Susan SG et al. The prevalence of domestic violence among women seeking abortion. *Obstetrics and Gynecology*, 1998, 91:1002-6.
[23] Evins G., Chescheir N. Prevalence of domestic violence among women seeking abortion services. *Women's Health Issues*, 1996, 6:204-10.
[24] Campbell H et al. Correlates of battering during pregnancy. *Research Nurse Health*, 1993, 15:219-26.

traditional cultural mores and taboos, which both normalize wife abuse and forbid discussion of that abuse. At an individual level, shame, guilt and fear of recrimination further silence any discussion of violence in the home. Therefore, most battering still remains hidden, undisclosed to neighbours, relatives, clinicians and researchers. However, in recent years, traditional taboos have begun to break down and domestic violence is slowly moving from being regarded as a totally private problem to being perceived as a public issue with social, as well as individual solutions. Gradually domestic violence is 'coming out of the closet' and its social implications are being recognized.

However, while the research on domestic violence against women is growing, it is still limited. We do know that, in 1984 in Shanghai, China, 6% of all female cases of serious injury or death were as a result of domestic violence. A survey by the National Women's Federation revealed that the prevalence of domestic violence against women was 30% in a sample of 27 million families studied in 1999[25]. Another survey on divorce in China revealed that 45.8% of women had reported domestic violence against themselves, and in 2000, a study on sexual coercion among 653 young adults showed that 15.6% of young adult women had become pregnant with an unwanted child because they had been sexually coerced and about 53% of young adults had experienced at least one episode of sexual coercion[26].

Health providers are often the first and sometimes the only professionals to whom an abused woman turns for help. They thus have a unique opportunity and responsibility to intervene. However, many fail to recognize the problem because they do not routinely inquire about, or document, abuse as the cause of their patients' symptoms, despite the fact that health practitioners see many victims of domestic violence in their clinical practices. Traditionally, health providers in China have not been trained in how to screen for domestic violence, or how to respond when domestic violence affects their patients. Consequently, the violence in a patient's life is often not addressed. According to the American Medical Association, "battered patients often present with repeated injuries, medical complaints and mental health problems, all of which result from living in an abusive situation. Medical care providers in all practice settings routinely see the consequences of domestic violence and abuse, but often fail to acknowledge their violent etiologies."[27]

There is a dearth of research on domestic violence against women related to pregnancy and there is therefore an urgent need to answer the following questions. What are the extent and forms of violence against pregnant women? What is the prevalence of abuse in the population of women who are seeking early pregnancy termination? Which populations (social class, education, ethnicity, geography, urban-rural) are most affected? Which factors are associated with violence against pregnant women? What is the impact on women's mental and physical health and the outcomes of their pregnancies? How do men perceive domestic violence? What is the level of health providers' knowledge about violence against pregnant women, and what are their attitudes and practices related to domestic violence?

STUDY OBJECTIVES

General objective

The broad objective of the study was to investigate the rates of domestic violence before, during and after pregnancy, the possible factors related to domestic violence, and the consequences of violence on the mental and physical health of mothers and infants.

Specific objectives

(1) To describe the prevalence and patterns of violent incidents against women before, during and after pregnancy, and among women who seek pregnancy termination;

(2) to identify the possible factors associated with violence before and during pregnancy and postpartum;

---

[25] China Says 'No' to Domestic Violence, www.english.peopledaily.com.cn, Wednesday, 27 November 2002.
[26] Cheng Yimin, Kang Baohua, Wang Tieyan, et al. Study on factors related to unintended sex. *Chinese Journal of Behavioral Medical Science*, 2000, 9(5):373-4.
[27] Salber P, Taliferro E. Physician's guide to intimate partner violence and abuse. Volcano, CA, Volcano Press, 1995.

(3) to understand victims' experiences and their perceptions related to gender roles and wife abuse;

(4) to understand men's perceptions related to gender roles and wife abuse; and

(5) to investigate health providers' knowledge, attitudes and practices regarding domestic violence.

CHAPTER 2.
LITERATURE REVIEW

This chapter reviews the findings from some previous studies. The review emphasizes the characteristics, risk factors and outcomes of domestic violence among pregnant women.

Domestic violence during pregnancy has been recognized as an important risk to the health of both the mother and the fetus or infant[28]. Previous studies have documented a rate of abuse during pregnancy of 5.5%-17%, depending on the population studied and the screening method used, and that the problem may be largely unreported to health care providers[29,30,31,32]. The 2005 WHO Multi-country Study found prevalence rates for physical violence against women varied from 1% in Japanese urban areas to 28% in a provincial town in Peru[33]. The study revealed that not all of the countries with very high overall levels of physical violence had correspondingly high levels of physical violence during pregnancy, suggesting that "in some settings violence during pregnancy is less accepted, even if violence against women is common". This lack of acceptability may also mean that violence during pregnancy is seriously underreported as it is a taboo even for women to admit to being abused while pregnant. Of the women who had been abused in pregnancy, the WHO study found that between 13% and 50% said that they had been "beaten for the first time during a pregnancy". Furthermore, of the pregnant women who had been abused before as well as during pregnancy, 8%-34% reported that "the violence got worse during pregnancy". There are some indications that violence during pregnancy may be a more prevalent problem than pregnancy-induced hypertension, gestational diabetes, or placenta previa, conditions for which pregnant women are routinely screened[34]. Susan and colleagues, as well as Evins, found that the prevalence rate of self-reported abuse in the population of women in early pregnancy seeking termination services was between 31% and 39.5%, and that women in abusive relationships were more likely to consider termination[35,36].

CHARACTERISTICS OF DOMESTIC VIOLENCE AGAINST PREGNANT WOMEN

1. Sociodemographic characteristics

The results of studies examining the sociodemographic factors contributing to domestic violence are ambiguous. Hilde found little difference between abused and non-abused pregnant women in terms of race, age, marital status, employment or educational status[37]. He did find, however, that women who reported abuse by a current or previous partner, or both, were more likely than non-abused women to report that their partners were unemployed. Another study found that, compared with non-abused

---

[28] *Op cit*. Ref 15.
[29] *Op cit*. Ref 16.
[30] *Op cit*. Ref 17.
[31] *Op cit*. Ref 18.
[32] Amaro H *et al*. Violence during pregnancy and substance use. *American Journal of Public Health*, 1990, 80:575-89.
[33] *Op cit*. Ref 2:65.
[34] *Op cit*. Ref 20.
[35] *Op cit*. Ref 22.
[36] *Op cit*. Ref 23.
[37] Hilde G et al. Physical abuse and low birth weight: a case-control study. *British Journal of Obstetrics and Gynaecology*, 1997, 104:1281-7.

women, women who had experienced abuse during pregnancy were of lower socioeconomic status, higher parity and more likely to be single[38]. Lynn's study found that having public insurance was associated with reduced levels of abuse in pregnancy[39].

Teenagers may be especially vulnerable to date rape, and teen pregnancies are sometimes the result of coercive sexual experiences. In previous studies, the rate of abuse reported by pregnant teens ranged from 21% to 31.6%[40,41,42]. Some have speculated that the female adolescent may be more vulnerable to violence because of female gender-role beliefs that her status is dependent on her attachment to a male, and her lack of experience in making decisions. In addition, pregnant adolescents who are exposed to violence appear to be at increased risk for substance abuse, inadequate prenatal care and poor birth outcomes. Indeed, the WHO Multi-country Study found that youth was a particular risk factor for violence. "With the exception of urban Japan city and Ethiopia province, younger ever-partnered women…aged 15-19 years were at higher risk of experiencing current physical or sexual violence or both, by an intimate partner"[43].

Paula's study in 1985 found that more abused women than control patients were in the lowest financial category or were receiving Medicaid assistance[44]. The same was true for the national crime survey data and other studies. In a group that included women who had noted past abuse but were no longer in an abusive relationship, the abused women were more likely to be divorced or separated than the control subjects. The WHO Multi-country Study reinforces those findings, indicating that, across all sites, "women who are separated or divorced generally reported a higher lifetime prevalence of all forms of violence than currently married women"[45]. This may reflect the fact that women who are divorced or separated feel more free to disclose past violence.

The WHO 2005 study also concurs with earlier research on the central role of poverty and low level of education as risk factors for both violators and survivors of domestic violence. However, the study notes that "the protective effect of education does not appear to start until women achieve the very highest levels of education (i.e. beyond secondary school)"[46]. However, it may be that women with very high levels of education are less willing to lose standing by disclosing violence in their families.

2. History of reproduction and pregnancy outcome

Studies show that abuse is a significant predictor of poor obstetric history, including low birth-weight, preterm delivery, miscarriage and fetal/neonatal death. One study in Sweden revealed that, of the 132 women answering a questionnaire on violence frequency, 32 reported threats, physical or sexual abuse postpartum[47]. In some studies, abuse has been associated significantly with low birth-weight[48,49,50]. For example, Parker's research in 1994 revealed that for the aggregate sample of 1203 women, abuse during pregnancy was a significant risk for low birth-weight and low maternal weight gain.

Battered women have also reported spontaneous abortions and stillbirths following episodes of battering. Furthermore, a 1996 study of women seeking pregnancy termination used a single screening interview and identified 31% of the women with a history of abuse[51]. Susan's' research in 1998 showed

---

[38] Paula J, Adams H. Physical abuses in pregnancy. *Obstetrics and gynecology*, 1985, 66(2): 185-90.
[39] Lynn BN, Jeffrey FP, Sally Z. Battering in pregnancy: an assessment of two screening methods. *Obstetrics and gynecology*, 1995, 85: (3) 321-5.
[40] *Op cit*. Ref 20.
[41] Parker, Barbara, et al. Physical and Emotional Abuse in Pregnancy: A Comparison of Adult and Teenage Women. *42 Nursing Research*, May/June 1993, 173-177.
[42] Mary AC, Nancy, Eric W. Effects of abuse on maternal complications and birth weight in adult and adolescent women. *Obstetrics and Gynecology*, 1998, 92:(4) 530-4.
[43] *Op cit*. Ref 2:32.
[44] *Op cit*. Ref 38.
[45] *Op cit*. Ref 2:33.
[46] *Ibid*.
[47] Hedin LW *et al*. Prevalence of physical and sexual abuse before and during pregnancy among Swedish couples. *Acta Obstetrics and Gynecology Scan*, 1999 Apr, 78(4): 310-5.
[48] *Op cit*. Ref 20.
[49] *Op cit*. Ref 47.
[50] Muhajarine N, D'Arcy C. Physical abuses during pregnancy: prevalence and risk factors. *Canadian Medical Association Journal*, 1999 Apr 6, 160(7): 1007-11.
[51] *Op cit*. Ref 23.

that the prevalence of self-reported abuse in the population was 39.5%, and that abused women may have different reasons for pregnancy termination than non-abused women[52]. Abused women may also be more likely to make the decision to abort without partner involvement.

3. Medical risk

Several studies show that abuse is associated significantly with inadequate prenatal care, poor prenatal weight gain, anaemia, first or second trimester bleeding, and infections[53,54,55]. In Mcfarlane's 1992 study, abused women were twice as likely as non-abused women to delay the start of prenatal care until the third trimester[56]. Cohen's survey revealed that between 67% and 83% of HIV-positive women in one clinic were still, or had been, in abusive relationships with men who refused to use barrier protection[57]. In one random population study, 45% of women with sexual problems and 47% of those with other gynecological complaints were battered women[58].

4. Mental illness

One study found that, compared with non-abused women, women who had experienced abuse during pregnancy were more likely to have a history of depression or other psychiatric symptoms[59]. In the same study, 25% of all women seen in the Emergency Department with psychiatric symptoms were battered women. The relationship between abuse and psychological dysfunction has major implications for women's mortality through increased risk of suicide. Studies from the United States of America have indicated that abused women are four to five times more likely to require psychiatric treatment and five times more likely to attempt suicide than non-battered women.

5. History of substance abuse

Abused women are also more likely to report alcohol abuse, and a trend in the data indicates that they might also have higher levels of illicit drug abuse. While a number of studies have found significant correlations between substance abuse and battering for both victims and perpetrators, it is clear that substance abuse does not always cause domestic violence[60,61]. As Carole points out, alcohol and drug abuse are likely to be consequences of the abuse or coping mechanisms, rather than purely causative factors[62].

HEALTH CONSEQUENCES OF DOMESTIC VIOLENCE AGAINST PREGNANT WOMEN

Many research studies have shown that domestic violence can cause adverse physical health events such as: injuries (from lacerations to fractures and internal organ injury); headaches; asthma; permanent disabilities; self-injurious behaviour (smoking, unprotected sex, alcohol and drug abuse); unwanted pregnancies; gynaecological problems; sexually transmitted infections, including HIV; pelvic inflammatory disease; chronic pelvic pain; and obstetrical manifestations of abuse, including miscarriages, spontaneous abortion, low birth-weight, multiple abortions, placental separation, rupture of the uterus and preterm labour[63]. It can also cause mental health outcomes, including depression, fear, anxiety, low self-esteem, sexual dysfunction, eating disorders, obsessive-compulsive disorder, posttraumatic stress disorder, fatal outcomes, suicide and homicide.

---

[52] *Op cit.* Ref 22.
[53] *Op cit.* Ref 20.
[54] *Op cit.* Ref 47.
[55] *Op cit.* Ref 50.
[56] *Op cit.* Ref 16.
[57] Cohen M *et al.* Domestic violence and childhood sexual abuse in HIV-infected women and women at risk for HIV. *American Journal of Public Health*, 2000, 90:560-565.
[58] Schei B, Bakkereig LS. Gynecological impact of sexual and physical abuse by spouse: a study of a random sample of Norwegian women. *British Journal of Obstetrics and Gynaecology*, 1989, 96:1379-83.
[59] Stark E, Flitcraft A. killing the beast within: woman battering and female suicide. *International Journal of Health Sciences*, 1995, 25(1): 43-64.
[60] Abbey BB et al. Drug abuse and other risk factors for physical abuse in pregnancy among white non-Hispanic, black, and Hispanic women. *American Journal of Obstetrics and Gynecology*, 1991, 164:1491-9.
[61] Kanto GK, Straus MA. Substance abuse as a precipitant of wife abuse victimization. *American Journal of Drug and Alcohol Abuse*, 1989, 15:178-89.
[62] *Op cit.* Ref 21.
[63] *Op cit.* Ref 20.

Witnessing domestic violence affects children in a variety of ways, and the effects are both short- and long-term[64]. Children may be physically, emotionally and cognitively damaged as a result of domestic violence. The negative effects of the perpetrator's abuse in interrupting childhood development can be seen in cognitive, psychological and physical symptoms such as: eating and sleeping disorders; mood-related disorders, such as depression and emotional neediness; over-compliance, clinging, withdrawal; aggressive acting out/destructive rages; detachment, avoidance, a fantasy family life; somatic complaints; finger biting, restlessness, shaking, stuttering; school problems; and suicide ideation.

DOMESTIC VIOLENCE SCREENING AND INTERVENTION

Lisa Moore suggests that every woman should be considered a possible victim of domestic violence[65]. Domestic violence occurs across all ethnic, cultural, religious and socioeconomic groups. The only consistent risk factor for abuse is being female[66]. Most women will not volunteer information about such abuse, but they will answer direct questions when they feel secure in the confidentiality of their answers. The literature suggests use of the following questions for domestic violence screening:

"Have you been hurt, threatened or frightened by someone who is close to you?"

"Do you fear for your safety or the safety of your children from a present or past partner?"

"Are you afraid of your partner or anyone else?"

"Has anyone hurt or threatened you during this pregnancy?"

"Have you been forced to perform sexual acts against your will?"

"What does your partner do when he/she is angry?"

Once a woman is identified as abused, the physician should provide necessary medical treatment, document the abuse, make appropriate referrals, and assist the patient in making an exit plan[67].

Health care interventions can occur at many levels. Primary prevention is designed to stop violence against women before it begins, thus averting health problems. Secondary prevention is aimed at ending existing violence early in the process and preventing further damage. Tertiary interventions are designed to end chronic violence and deal with the short- and long-term consequences of that violence, including rehabilitation. It is necessary to train health providers who are unfamiliar with the issues surrounding violence against women so that they can provide services whenever needed.

CONCLUSIONS

Domestic violence against pregnant women has begun to receive increased attention in the international arena as a human rights issue and, more recently, as a public health concern. Violence against pregnant women constitutes a serious health risk to pregnant women and their children. Health care providers can play an important role in a coordinated community response to domestic violence by: acting in ways that increase the safety of the victim and her children; supporting victims in making their own decisions about their lives; holding the perpetrators, not the victims, responsible for domestic violence; and helping to rehabilitate those who have suffered chronic violence.

---

[64] Warshaw C, Ganley AL eds. Improving the health care response to domestic violence: a resource manual for health care providers. San Francisco, Family Violence Prevention Fund, 1998.
[65] Moore LL. Dangerous intimacies: toward a Sapphic history of the British novel. Duke university Press, 1997.
[66] Holtz K. A practical approach to clients who are survivors of childhood sexual abuse. *Journal of Nurse-Midwifery*, 1994, 39(1): 13-18.
[67] *Op cit.* Ref 65.

Chapter 3. Methodology

RESEARCH DESIGN

In order to achieve all the objectives of the study, both quantitative and qualitative research techniques were employed. The primary research method was a quantitative study, while a qualitative study (in-depth interviews, focus group discussions) was used as a supplementary method. A cross-sectional study was used in the quantitative research.

RESEARCH SITES AND TIME PERIOD

The survey was conducted in Tianjing, Liaoning, Henan and Shannxi provinces from November 2001 to February 2002. Seven cities and 32 communities were involved.

RESEARCH METHODS

1. Community-based survey on women who had delivered a baby within 6-18 months

(a) Target population:

The target population was women who had children aged from 6 to 18 months, had resided in the sampling area for at least one year and were registered in the city.

(b) Sample size:

The appropriate sample size was assigned on the basis of a 95% confidence level. The estimated prevalence rate of domestic violence during pregnancy was 4%. Therefore, the sample size was 12 000. A stratified sampling technique was used to select the sample. Thirty-two communities were randomly selected in four study areas, and 375 women were interviewed in each community. Finally, 12 044 women who had babies aged 6-18 months were interviewed.

(c) Data collection:

All women whose babies had been registered at an immunization clinic in the research areas were interviewed, either in the immunization clinic or at home.

2. Clinic-based study on women seeking abortions

(a) Target population:

The target population was women seeking pregnancy terminations in family planning clinics, who had resided in the sampling area for at least one year and who were registered in the city.

(b) Sample size:

The appropriate sample size was assigned on the basis of a 95% confidence level. The estimated prevalence rate of domestic violence in the population of women seeking pregnancy terminations was 15%. Therefore, the sample size was 1200. A total of 150 cases were collected in each city. Finally, 1215 women who were seeking abortions were interviewed.

(c) Data collection:

Women were recruited consecutively in family planning departments in women's and children's hospitals in Tianjing, Liaoning, Henan and Shaanxi.

3. In-depth interviews with abused women who had delivered babies within 6-18 months

After a general questionnaire was administered to explore domestic violence against women before, during and after pregnancy, a sample of abused women was recruited for interview by a maternal and child health worker. In-depth interviews were conducted by one researcher and lasted between one and two hours for each case. A total of 12 abused women were interviewed in depth.

4. Focus group discussion with men with children under five years of age

Each man was recruited from paediatric departments while he was seeing a doctor for his child. One focus group discussion was conducted with men in each of the seven cities selected for the study.

5. Survey on health providers' knowledge, attitudes and practices regarding to domestic violence.

All the health providers who were attending a training course on reproductive health were recruited, giving a total of 139.

RESEARCH INSTRUMENTS

The following methods were used to collect the data for the study:

1. Structured questionnaire

A structured questionnaire was used as the major research tool to collect information on the prevalence rate of domestic violence against women who had babies aged 6-18 months and women who were seeking pregnancy termination, and to identify possible factors related to domestic violence. The structured interview questionnaire incorporated key variables associated with domestic violence, as identified in the literature review. It consisted of eight sections, each section concentrating on the following specific issues:

(a) the sociodemographic characteristics of each studied woman and her partner, as well as substance abuse;

(b) the history of reproduction, pregnancy outcome, and the physical impact of pregnancy on the woman;

(c) psychological problems (Self-rating Depression Scale);

(d) the respondent's attitude toward domestic violence and gender roles;

(e) lifetime experience of domestic violence;

(f) relationship with partner;

(g) the domestic violence situation in the family; and

(h) the respondent's response to domestic violence.

2. In-depth interview guidelines

The women were asked open-ended questions about the positive and negative aspects of their relationships with their husbands. They were also asked to recount the worst and most recent incidents of violence in their relationships before, during and after pregnancy. Interviews were semi-structured; interviewers were instructed to cover the topics suggested by the guiding questions and to pursue topics raised by the participants.

3. Focus group discussion guidelines

The focus group discussion guidelines included: (1) The standard of "a good husband"; (2) The man's role in the family; (3) The standard of "a good wife"; (4) The woman's role in the family; (5) Attitudes towards gender roles; and (6) Attitudes towards gender-related violence.

4. **Structured questionnaire on health providers' knowledge, attitudes and practices regarding domestic violence**

The questionnaire included three parts: sociodemographic characteristics, attitude towards domestic violence, and health provider's practices.

TRAINING OF INTERVIEWERS

A training workshop on screening, assessment and intervention methods for domestic violence and methods of conducting surveys on domestic violence was held from 28 October to 2 November 2001 in Beijing. Forty-four maternal and child health workers from Tianjing, Henan, Shaanxi and Liaoning took part in the training workshop and were subsequently involved in the project.

OPERATIONAL DEFINITIONS

1. **Domestic violence** refers to a pattern of assault or coercive behaviour, including physical, sexual and psychological attacks by intimate partners.

    Physical abuse (PHYA) was measured by any of the following:

    - Beat or pushed you, but without trauma or persistent pain or limited movement in some parts of your body.
    - Hit you with his fist, kicked or cut you, with persistent pain or limited movement in some parts of your body.
    - Beat you up seriously, with contusion, burn or fracture.
    - Head or viscera trauma, with permanent injury.
    - Injured you with tools or a weapon.

    Sexual abuse (SEXA) was measured by following:

    - Continuously insisted that you had sexual intercourse.
    - Threatened you to have sexual intercourse, by any means.
    - Physically forced you to have sexual intercourse.
    - Tied you with a rope or something else in order to force you to have sexual intercourse.
    - Hit you first, then forced you to have sexual intercourse.

    Psychological abuse (PSYA) was measured by following:

    - Often insulted you or made you feel bad.
    - Often humiliated you in front of other people.
    - Threatened to divorce or leave you.
    - Threatened to hit you or someone else you care about.
    - Took something with intent to hit you or scare you.

2. **History of reproduction** refers to times of gestation and whether the woman had a history of miscarriage, a low-birth-weight baby, a pre-term delivery, and/or fetal/neonatal death etc., the number of abortions and any gynaecological disease.

3. **Psychological problems** within one week refer to the woman's self-reported symptoms and were measured by using the Self-rating Depression Scale.

4. **Medical complications** refer to whether the woman had any maternal complications, such as anaemia

5. **Pregnancy outcome** refers to whether the woman had poor obstetric outcomes such as a low-birth-weight baby, a premature delivery, a miscarriage, and/or fetal/neonatal death etc.

6. **Substance abuse** refers to the woman smoking or abusing alcohol or other drugs.

7. **Lifetime experience** refers to whether the woman knew about domestic violence or had experienced it throughout her life.

8. **Relationship with partner** refers to whether the woman's partner treated her badly, according to eight questions.

DATA PROCESSING AND ANALYSIS

Data were double-entered into a computerized database using Epi Info 6.0 and data analysis was carried out using SPSS/PC V10.0 for Windows. The entered data were screened and checked logistically for consistency before data analysis. Domestic violence was examined as a dichotomy (0 for no domestic violence, 1 for ever domestic violence), and the significance of association with the domestic violence variable was examined using the χ^2, T test statistic. The Fisher exact test was used for variables with small expected cell frequencies. The criterion for statistical significance was set at $P < 0.05$. A multivariate logistic regression model was used to identify factors associated with domestic violence, poor obstetric outcome and postnatal depression. The criterion for statistical significance was set at $P < 0.05$.

In-depth interviews and focus group discussions were recoded and transcribed. The analysis steps were as follows: data sorting, data coding and logical analysis.

ETHICAL CONSIDERATIONS

All data were collected with the informed oral consent of the respondents in private spaces free from the influence of others. The respondents were reassured that their interviews were confidential and that the study results would be reported anonymously. Respondents were fully informed of the purpose of the study and any benefits that would result from it. They were allowed to withdraw if they did not wish to be interviewed after the researcher had explained the purpose of the study. During the survey and interviews, all respondents were treated with respect and were thanked for their contributions to the study. No data which identify the individuals interviewed will be revealed to anyone other than the researchers, and all raw data will remain stored in locked filing cabinets for five years after the study is completed, after which time it will be shredded.

CHAPTER 4.
DOMESTIC VIOLENCE AGAINST WOMEN BEFORE, DURING AND AFTER PREGNANCY

This chapter is divided into two parts. The first part presents the results, while the second discusses those results. The first part is divided into five sections: (1) General description of the women's characteristics; (2) Domestic violence situation (before, during and after pregnancy); (3) Factors associated with domestic violence; (4) Effects of abuse on women's reproductive health; and (5) Results of in-depth interviews with abused women.

RESULTS

The study consisted of a survey of 12 044 women in seven northern cities of China who had delivered babies in the previous 6-18 months. The survey was followed by in-depth interviews with a sample of those women identified as having been exposed to intimate partner abuse.

1. Women's characteristics

   1.1 Sociodemographic characteristics of the women and their spouses

   (a) Age

   The ages of the women ranged from 19-45 years, with a mean of 27.6 years. The ages of the women's husbands ranged from 20-57 years, with a mean of 29.6 years. Nearly three-quarters (73.8%) of the women were younger than their husbands.

   (b) Education

   The mean number of years of schooling for the women was 12.2, while it was 12.7 for their husbands. More than half (56.7%) of the women had attained the same level of education as their husbands. Nearly one-third (30.9%) of the women had education levels that were lower than their husbands. Over one-tenth (12.4%) of the women had an education level higher than their husbands.

   (c) Occupation

   Before their most recent pregnancy, the first three leading occupations of the women were: worker (29.1%), officer (19.5%) and professional technician (12.4%). However, after pregnancy, the first three leading occupation were unemployed (24.6%), worker (23.9%) and officer (19.1%). For the husbands, the first three leading occupations were: worker (30.1%), officer (23.6%) and professional technician (13.6%). When the occupations were classified into white- or blue-collar workers, the results showed that, before delivery, 44.5% of the women were white-collar workers; while after delivery, 40.6% of the women were white-collar workers. Just over half of the husbands (50.5%) were white-collar workers.

   (d) Duration of marriage

   The lengths of the women's marriages ranged from 1-20 years, with a mean of 3.2, while those of their husbands ranged from 1 to 33 years, with a mean of 3.3. Marital status was also classified into stable (98.8%) (including first marriage) and unstable (1.2%) (including divorced, separated and remarried).

   (e) Income

   Before pregnancy, slightly more than one-fifth (21.6%) of the women had received a monthly income of less than 300 Yuan (approximately US$ 37.00), while just under half (47.8%) had received an income of 301-800 Yuan. Less than one-third (30.6%) of the women had received an income higher than 800 Yuan (approximately US$ 100.00). However, after delivery, the level of the women's incomes decreased: 36.8% of them had a monthly income of less than 300 Yuan, 36.3% had a monthly income of 301-800 Yuan and 26.8% had a monthly income higher than 800 Yuan.

   The husbands' incomes presented a very different pattern to that of their wives. Only 7.6% of the men had a monthly income of less than 300 Yuan, 34.4% had a monthly income of 301-800 Yuan, and most (58.0%) of them had a monthly income higher than 800 Yuan. In most cases (52.7%), the women's incomes were lower than their husbands' incomes. After delivery, the percentage of women earning substantially less than their husbands grew to 59.0%.

(f) Types of family

More than half (64.1%) of the women lived in a nuclear family, 35.2% of them lived in an extended family, while 0.6% of them lived alone.

(g) Substance abuse

There were low levels of reported substance use and abuse among the women in the study. Only 2.6% of the women were smokers, 11.5% of them were alcohol users and 0.6% of them reported that they were illicit drug users.

The husbands' levels of reported substance use and abuse were much higher: 68.4% of them were smokers, 75% of them were alcohol users, but only 0.8% of them reported that they were illicit drug users.

(h) Emotion after childbirth

Most of the family members (93.5% of the women, 95% of the husbands and 90.2% of the parents-in-law) reported being happy after the baby was born.

In summary, the women interviewed were young and newly married. Although the women's levels of education were similar with their husbands', they suffered lower socioeconomic conditions in terms of occupation and income. After delivery, the women's socioeconomic conditions became worse.

1.2   Attitudes towards gender roles

It is noteworthy that most of the women did not know what their rights were. Therefore, most of their answers were "uncertain" (see Table 1).

Table 1. Attitudes towards gender roles

	Agree (%)	Disagree (%)	Uncertain (%)
1. A good wife should obey her husband even if she disagrees with his thoughts or actions.	902 (7.5)	1567 (13.0)	9573 (79.5)
2. A man should show his wife/partner that he is the head of the family.	2139 (17.8)	1377 (11.4)	8526 (70.8)
3. A woman should be able to choose her own friends even if her husband disapproves.	1806 (15.0)	1847 (15.3)	8389 (69.7)
4. It is a wife's obligation to have sex with her husband even if she is unwilling.	941 (7.8)	1302 (10.8)	9797 (81.4)
5. In your opinion, a man has a rational reason to hit his wife when:			
(a) she does not complete her housekeeping to his satisfaction;	187 (1.6)	218 (1.8)	11637 (96.6)
(b) she disobeys him;	167 (1.4)	235 (2.0)	11640 (96.6)
(c) she refuses to have sexual activities with him;	185 (1.5)	345 (2.9)	11512 (95.6)
(d) she asks him whether he has other girlfriends; or	292 (2.4)	482 (4.0)	11268 (93.6)
(e) he suspects that she is unfaithful.	702 (5.8)	757 (6.3)	10583 (87.9)

1.3   Attitudes towards domestic violence

In answer to the statement: "Family problems should only be discussed with family members", slightly more than one-third (38.7%) of the women agreed; one-fifth (20.1%) of them did not agree and 41.2% of them were not sure. Regarding attitudes towards the statement: "If a man mistreats his wife, others outside the family should intervene", only 11.8% of the women agreed and 5.8% of them did not agree. However, most of them (82.4%) were not sure.

If the women were abused, they said they would first seek help from family members (38.3%) or friends (32.2%), but 16.9% said that they would not tell anyone. The second choice was family members (27.8%), friends (21.3%) and women's organizations (13.1%). The third choice was women's organizations (17.8%), colleagues (13.8%) and the police (10.8%)

1.4 Life experience

Nearly one-third (30.5%) of the women knew other women that were being battered by their husbands. More than one-tenth (13.4%) of them had witnessed their mothers being battered by their fathers, and 7.1% of them knew that their mothers-in-law were being battered by their fathers-in-law.

1.5 Relationship with husband

Regarding the relationship between couples: 13.6% of the women said that they were afraid of their husbands; fewer than one-third (30.4%) of them had never, or seldom, quarreled with their husbands; 10.6% of the women were ignored by their husbands frequently, while 15.0% were ignored sometimes; 4.8% of the women said that their husbands harmed their pets or items in the house; 20% of the women said that their husbands would be angry if they talked with other men; 7.7% of the husbands put pressure on their wives to deliver boys; 24.3% of the women often, or sometimes, sought agreement from their husbands before going to prenatal check-ups; 10.2% of the women said that their husbands did not like to give them money, sometimes or frequently, when they needed it.

1.6 Reproductive history

The majority (63.4%) of the women interviewed were pregnant for the first time, and for 97.1% of them it was their first delivery. One-tenth (10.2%) of the women had a history of spontaneous abortion. Slightly more than one-third (38.2%) of them had a history of abortion(s).

The mean time for the first prenatal check-up was 11.18±4.5 weeks. Only slightly more than one-third (35.5%) started prenatal check-ups in the first trimester. The mean number of prenatal check-ups was 9.63±3.33 visits. The women's poor obstetric histories are shown in Table 2.

Table 2. Obstetric history

	Never (%)	In latest pregnant (%)	In the previous pregnancy (%)	In both the latest and previous pregnancy(%)
Vaginal bleeding	10228 (84.9)	1161 (9.6)	544 (4.5)	110 (0.9)
Pre-term delivery	11675 (97.0)	340 (2.8)	25 (0.2)	1 (0.0)
Intrauterine growth retardation	11965 (99.3)	53 (0.4)	25 (0.2)	1 (0.0)
Placenta abruption	12012 (99.8)	24 (0.2)	6 (0.0)	0
Still-birth	11965 (99.3)	21 (0.2)	57 (0.5)	1 (0.0)
Anaemia	10593 (88.0)	1358 (11.3)	51 (0.4)	39 (0.3)
Neonatal death	12008 (99.7)	12 (0.1)	22 (0.2)	0
Premature rupture of membranes	11675 (97.0)	353 (2.9)	10 (0.1)	3 (0.0)

1.7 Prevalence of depression

The Self-rating Depression Scale was used to evaluate the women's depression within one week of delivery. The results show that the depression scale ranged from 20 to 72, with a mean of 33.45±7.72. Prevalence of depression was 20.9%, with light depression in 15.5% of cases, medium depression in 4.7% and severe depression in 0.7%.

1.8 Babies' health status

Most (92.9%) of the neonates' birth weights were between 2500g~4000g. The rate of low birth-weight was 1.7% Cwhile 5.4% were bigger than 4000g. The morbidity rate for neonates was 2.5%.

All women who had a baby aged older than one year were asked several questions about the infant's 'attack' behaviour, emotions, adaptability and withdrawal behaviour. For the 'attack' behaviour, the scale ranged from 2 to 6, with a mean of 2.92±1.04. The higher the score, the higher the level of 'attack' behaviour. The emotional scale ranged from 4 to12, with a mean of 6.37±1.57. The higher the score on the emotional scale, the higher the passivity. The adaptability scale ranged from 2 to 6, with a mean of 3.92±1.01. The higher the score on the adaptability scale, the lower the level of adaptability. The scale of withdrawal behavior ranged from 1 to 3, with a mean of 2.42±0.71. The lower the score on this scale, the higher the level of withdrawal.

2. Domestic violence situation

2.1 Prevalence of domestic violence in total (domestic violence in any of the three periods) before, during and after pregnancy

The results (Table 3) show that the total prevalence rate of domestic violence (DVT) across all periods (before, during and after pregnancy) was 12.6%. The prevalence rate for psychological abuse (PSYA) was 3.5%, for sexual abuse (SEXA) 8.0%, and for physical abuse (PHYA) 5.6%. The results also reveal the lowest rate of domestic violence was for domestic violence during pregnancy (DVDP). The prevalence rate was 9.1% for domestic violence before pregnancy (DVBP), 4.3% for domestic violence during pregnancy (DVDP), and 8.3% for domestic violence after pregnancy (DVAP). SEXA had the highest prevalence rate during all periods. (see also Figure 1).

Table 3. Prevalence of domestic violence

	Total (%)	PSYA (%)	SEXA (%)	PHYA (%)
DVBP	1093 (9.1)	232 (1.9)	704 (5.8)	473 (3.9)
DVDP	522 (4.3)	182 (1.5)	333 (2.8)	129 (1.1)
DVAP	998 (8.3)	305 (2.5)	593 (4.9)	387 (3.2)
DVT	1518 (12.6)	426 (3.5)	964 (8.0)	670 (5.6)

Figure 1. Prevalence of domestic violence

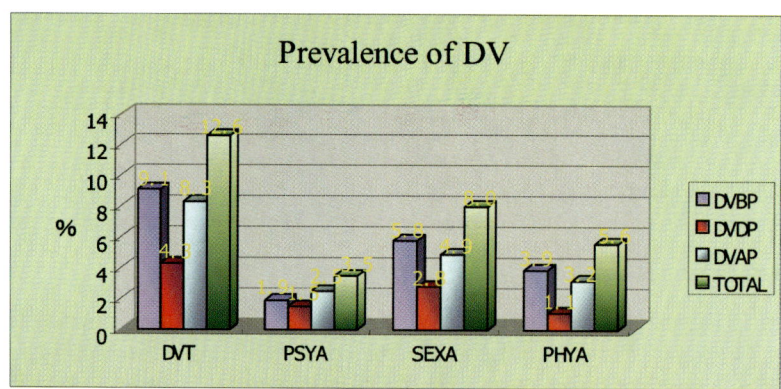

The results show that Shaanxi Province had the highest DVT, DVBP, DVDP and DVAP rates in the study (see Table 4).

Table 4. Domestic violence by province

Province (total cases)	DVT N (%)	DVBP N (%)	DVDP N (%)	DVAP N (%)
Henan (2996)	418 (14.0)	343 (11.4)	140 (4.7)	248 (8.3)
Liaoning (3008)	316 (10.5)	232 (7.7)	110 (3.7)	202 (6.7)
Shaanxi (3015)	559 (18.5)	371 (12.3)	195 (6.5)	381 (12.6)
Tianjin (3025)	225 (7.4)	147 (4.9)	77 (2.5)	167 (5.5)

2.2 Domestic violence by period

The results show low prevalence rates for cases where (1) domestic violence occurred only during pregnancy, (2) domestic violence occurred before and during pregnancy, but not after pregnancy, and (3) domestic violence occurred during and after pregnancy. (see Table 5 and Figure 2).

Table 5. Domestic violence by period

	Number of cases	Percentage (%)	Prevalence (%)
DVBP only	392	25.8	3.2
DVDP only	70	4.6	0.6
DVAP only	298	19.6	2.5
DVBP+DVDP	58	3.8	0.5
DVBP+DVAP	306	20.2	2.5
DVDP+DVAP	57	3.8	0.5
DVBP+DVDP+DVAP	337	22.2	2.8

Figure 2. Domestic violence by period

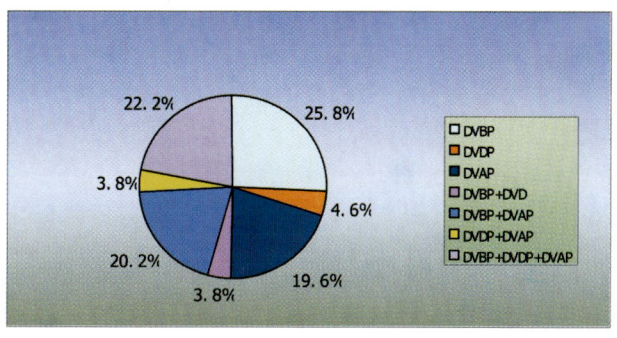

2.3 Pattern of domestic violence before, during and after pregnancy

DVBP was a strong risk factor for DVDP and DVAP, and domestic violence during a previous period was a strong risk factor for subsequent violence (see Figure 4). A strong, significant association was found between DVBP and DVDP (OR, 48.23 C95% CI,38.73-60.10) and there was also a strong, significant association between DVDP and DVAP (OR, 55.64 C95% CI, 44.61-69.44) and between DVBP and DVAP (OR, 42.65 C 95% CI,36.22-50.23). For those who recorded both DVBP and DVDP, the probability of having DVAP was very high (OR,96.59 C95% CI, 71.66-130.44). Only 2.5% of all the women had experienced domestic violence for the first time after delivery (i.e., they were abused after delivery, but not before or during pregnancy). Furthermore, the absence of DVBP and DVDP was a strong protective factor against DVAP (OR, 0.02; 95% CI, 0.02-0.02)

2.4 Types of domestic violence

As for the type of domestic violence, many (41.7%) of them were SEXA, one-tenth (10.5%) were PSYA only and one-fifth (19.8%) were PHYA only. The others were mixed PSHA, SEXA and PHYA (see Table 6 and Figure 3).

There were also strong associations among PSYA, SEXA, and PHYA (P<0.01). For example, between PSYA and PHYA (r≈0.367).

Table 6. Types of domestic violence

	Number	(%)
PSYA only	160	10.5
SEXA only	633	41.7
PHYA only	300	19.8
PSYA+SEXA	55	3.6
PSYA+PHYA	94	6.2
SEXA+PHYA	159	10.5
PSYA+SXEA+PHYA	117	7.7

Figure 3. Types of domestic violence

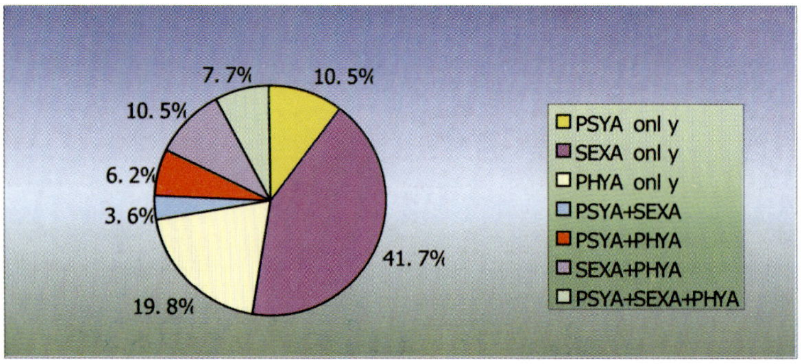

2.5 Frequency of domestic violence

The results in Table 7 show that in more than 50% of cases, domestic violence happened only once or twice. However, many domestic violence incidents were recurrent, indicating a long period of suffering.

Table 7. Frequency of domestic violence

	DVT (1518)				DVBP (1093)				DVDP (522)				DVAP (998)			
	DVT	PSYA	SEXA	PHYA	DVBP	PSYA	SEXA	PHYA	DVDP	PSYA	SEXA	PHYA	DVAP	PSYA	SEXA	PHYA
1-2	555 (36.6)	174 (40.8)	388 (40.2)	342 (51.0)	567 (51.9)	126 (54.3)	413 (58.7)	310 (65.5)	334 (64.0)	106 (58.2)	243 (73.0)	92 (71.3)	529 (53.0)	159 (52.1)	340 (57.3)	254 (65.6)
3-9	685 (45.1)	157 (36.9)	451 (46.8)	273 (40.8)	430 (39.3)	80 (34.5)	256 (36.4)	145 (30.7)	144 (27.6)	56 (30.8)	81 (24.3)	28 (21.7)	347 (34.8)	98 (32.1)	216 (36.4)	114 (29.5)
>=10	278 (18.3)	95 (22.3)	125 (13.0)	55 (8.2)	96 (8.8)	26 (11.2)	35 (4.9)	18 (3.8)	44 (8.4)	20 (11.0)	9 (2.7)	9 (7.0)	122 (12.2)	48 (15.8)	37 (6.3)	19 (4.9)

Figure 4. Patterns of domestic violence before, during and after pregnancy in women in Northern China, 2002

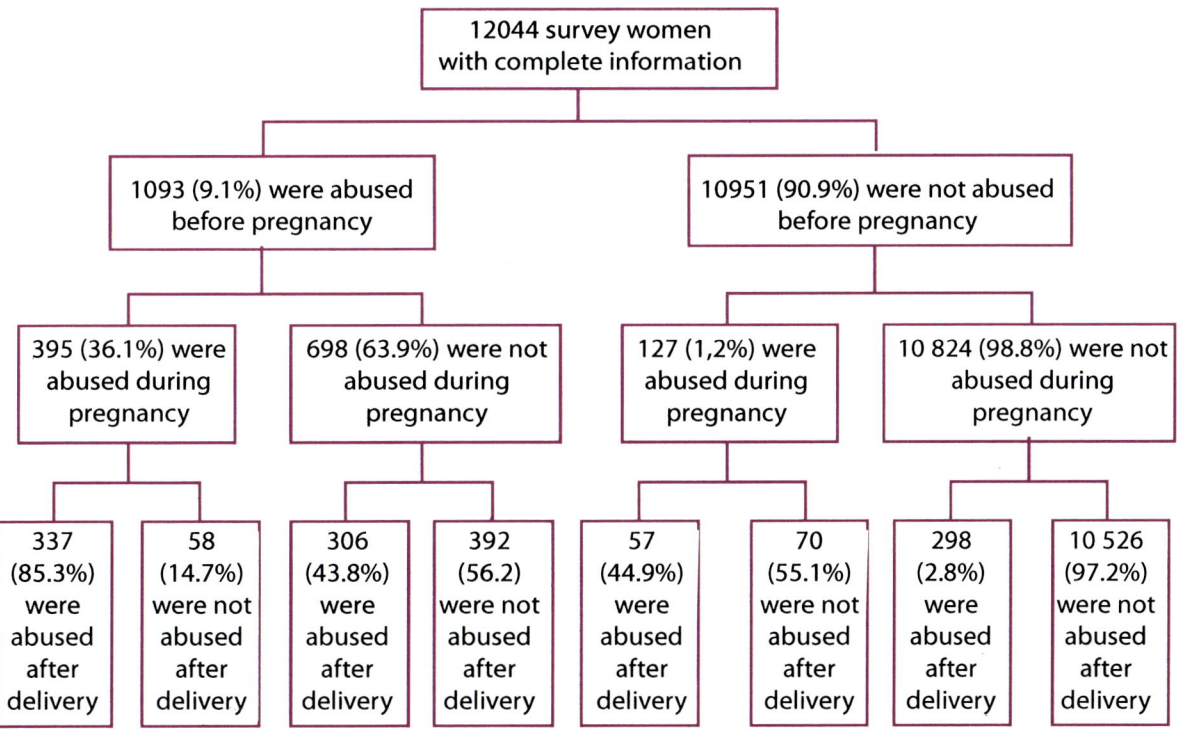

2.6 Severity of domestic violence

Table 8 shows the severity of domestic violence, by type. Whether PSYA, SEXA or PHYA, most of the abuse was not reported as severe.

Table 8. Severity of domestic violence by ty

	DVT (%)	DVBP (%)	DVDP (%)	DVAP (%)
(One woman may have suffered more than one type of abuse, so the total is not 100%.)				
PSYA				
1. Often insulted you or made you feel bad	306(71.8)	169(72.8)	130(71.4)	204(58.3)
2. Often humiliated you in front of other people	88(20.7)	32(13.8)	31(17.0)	60(17.1)
3. Threatened to divorce or leave you	123(28.9)	43(18.5)	40(22.0)	86(24.6)
4. Threatened to hit you or someone else you care about	89(20.9)	43(18.5)	35(19.3)	55(15.7)
5. Took something with intent to hit or scare you	183(43.0)	81(34.9)	53(29.1)	130(37.1)
SEXA				
1. Continuously insisted you have sexual intercourse	924(95.9)	670(95.2)	315(94.6)	558(94.1)
2. Threatened you to have sexual intercourse, by any means	76(7.9)	61(8.7)	40(12.0)	45(7.6)
3. Physically forced you to have sexual intercourse	130(13.5)	87(12.4)	45(13.5)	87(14.7)
4. Tied you with rope or something else in order to force you to have sexual intercourse	22(2.3)	19(2.7)	17(5.1)	19(3.2)
5. Hit you first, then forced you to have sexual intercourse	51(5.3)	40(5.7)	24(7.2)	34(5.7)
PHYA				
1. Beat or pushed you but without trauma or persistent pain or limited movement in some parts of your body	648(96.7)	461(97.5)	113(87.6)	362(93.6)
2. Hit you with fists, kicked or cut you, with persistent pain or limited movement in some parts of your body	116(17.3)	64(13.5)	34(26.4)	74(19.1)
3. Beat you up, with seriously contusions burn or fracture	13(1.9)	10(2.1)	9(7.0)	10(2.6)
4. Head or viscera trauma, permanent injury	14(2.1)	9(1.9)	8(6.2)	9(2.3)
5. Injured you with tools or a weapon	20(3.0)	14(3.0)	9(7.0)	12(3.1)
6. Hit your abdomen	44(6.6)	23(4.9)	16(12.4)	29(7.5)

2.7 Reasons for physical abuse

The most frequent reasons for abuse from the women's perception were: no special reason, after he was drunk, conflict between in-laws, dissatisfaction with his work, or the wife being disobedient towards her husband.

2.8 Women's actions after abuse

Only one-tenth (11.2%) of the women never hit back after being abused, and nearly half (44.6%) hit back every time. After abuse, the most frequent action of the abused women was not to tell anyone, family members or friends.

Thus, domestic violence happens before, during and after delivery. Compared with DVBP and DVAP, the prevalence of DVDP was lower in the area studied. DVBP is a strong risk factor for DVDP and DVAP, and domestic violence during a previous period is a strong risk factor for subsequent domestic violence. The types of domestic violence covered PSYA, SEXA and PHYA. SEXA was the most prevalent in the study. There were associations between PSYA, SEXA, and PHYA. Most of the abuse was not reported as severe.

3. Factors associated with domestic violence

3.1 Sociodemographic factors affecting the prevalence of domestic violence

(a) Women's sociodemographic status

The results show that abused women were more likely to have a lower level of education, have longer marriages, be blue-collar workers, have lower incomes, be in unstable marriages, live in extended families or alone, and be smokers or alcohol users ($p<0.05$). However, there appeared to be no significant relationship between domestic violence and a woman's age, or a history of illicit drug abuse (see Table 9).

Table 9. Women's sociodemographic status as a factor in domestic violence

	Abused (%)	Non-abused (%)	P
Age			>0.05
>30	1318 (86.8)	9302 (88.4)	
31<	200 (13.2)	1224 (11.6)	
Educational level			<0.001
Primary	40 (2.6)	142 (1.3)	
Junior high	338 (22.3)	2122 (20.2)	
Senior high	620 (40.9)	4246 (40.4)	
College or above	520 (34.2)	4016 (38.1)	
Years of marriage			<0.01
1 or more	1362 (89.7)	9688 (92.0)	
5 or more	130 (8.6)	691 (6.6)	
11 or more	26 (1.7)	146 (1.4)	
Occupation before pregnancy			<0.001
Blue-collar worker	921 (60.7)	5759 (54.7)	
White-collar worker	597 (39.3)	4767 (45.3)	
Occupation after pregnancy			<0.001
Blue-collar worker	997 (65.7)	6177 (58.7)	
White-collar worker	521 (34.3)	4348 (41.3)	
Income before pregnancy (Yuan)			<0.001
>300	352 (23.2)	2247 (21.3)	
301-800	819 (54.0)	4944 (47.0)	
801<	347 (22.9)	3335 (31.7)	
Income after pregnancy (Yuan)			<0.001
>300	618 (40.7)	3813 (36.2)	
301-800	594 (39.1)	3792 (36.0)	
801<	306 (20.2)	2921 (27.8)	

Table 9. Women's sociodemographic status as a factor in domestic violence (cont...)

	Abused (%)	Non-abused (i%)	P
Marital status			<0.001
Stable	1483 (97.7)	10402 (98.9)	
Unstable	35 (2.3)	114 (1.1)	
Type of family			<0.001
Nuclear	917 (60.4)	6807 (64.6)	
Extended	582 (38.3)	3661 (34.8)	
Alone	19 (1.3)	58 (0.6)	
Smoker			<0.001
No	1455 (95.8)	10276 (97.6)	
Yes	63 (4.2)	250 (2.4)	
Alcohol user			<0.001
No	1255 (82.7)	9407 (89.4)	
Sometimes	232 (15.3)	972 (9.2)	
Frequently	31 (2.0)	146 (1.4)	
Illicit drug user			>0.05
No	1504 (99.1)	10466 (99.4)	
Yes	14 (0.9)	60 (0.6)	

(b) Spouses' sociodemographic characteristics

The perpetrators of abuse, the women's spouses, were more likely to be older, have been married longer, have a lower level of education, be blue-collar workers, have lower incomes, and be smokers, alcohol users and illicit drug users (p<0.05) (see Table 10).

Table 10. Spouses' sociodemographic status as a factor in domestic violence

	Abused (%)	Non-abused(%)	P
Age			<0.01
>30	998 (65.7)	7361 (69.9)	
31-40	502 (33.1)	3043 (28.9)	
41<	18 (1.2)	122 (1.2)	
Years of marriage			=0.001
1 or more	1349 (88.9)	9653 (91.7)	
5 or more	135 (8.9)	702 (6.7)	
11 or more	34 (2.2)	171 (1.6)	
Educational level			<0.001
Primary	25 (1.6)	94 (0.9)	
Junior high	302 (19.9)	1734 (16.5)	
Senior high	552 (36.4)	3860 (36.6)	
College or above	639 (42.1)	4838 (46.0)	
Occupation	<0.001		
Blue-collar	854 (56.3)	5105 (48.5)	
White-collar	664 (43.7)	5419 (51.5)	
Income (Yuan)			<0.001
>300	136 (9.0)	781 (7.4)	
301-800	602 (39.7)	3536 (33.6)	
801<	780 (51.3)	6209 (59.0)	
Smoker			<0.001
No	387 (25.5)	3416 (32.5)	
Yes	1131 (74.5)	7109 (67.5)	
Alcohol user			<0.001
No	318 (20.9)	2700 (25.7)	
Sometimes	715 (47.1)	5054 (48.0)	
Frequently	485 (32.0)	2772 (26.3)	
Illicit drug user			<0.01
No	1497 (98.6)	10451 (99.3)	
Yes	21 (1.4)	75 (0.7)	

It was also found that those spouses who were younger than their female partners, and had a lower level of education, were more likely to be perpetrators of abuse (see Table 11).

Table 11. Differences between couples as a factor in domestic violence

	Abused (%)	Non-abused (%)	P
Age			=0.001
Husband younger	136 (9.0)	741 (7.0)	
Same	240 (15.8)	2036 (19.4)	
Husband older	1142 (75.2)	7749 (73.6)	
Educational level			<0.05
Husband lower	219 (14.4)	1279 (12.2)	
Same	832 (54.8)	5992 (56.9)	
Husband higher	467 (30.8)	3255 (30.9)	

3.2 Women's attitudes towards domestic violence

Women's attitudes towards the following two statements were analysed: (1) "Family problems should only be discussed with members of the family"; and (2) "If a man mistreats his wife, others outside the family should intervene".

Those women who believed that domestic violence was a private affair and that outsiders should not intervene were less likely to be abused ($p<0.05$) or, a more realistic explanation, were less likely to report abuse.

3.3 Women's attitudes towards gender roles and domestic violence

The results show that those women who were aware of their rights were less likely to be abused ($p<0.001$). However, the instrument measuring attitude towards gender roles was not an appropriate or sensitive enough measure of the women's understanding of their gender rights, as the majority of the women answered "uncertain' to all questions.

3.4 Life experience

A woman who knew someone around her was being hit by her husband, whose mother was being hit by her father, or whose mother-in-law was being hit by her father-in-law was more likely to be abused ($p<0.001$) (see Table 12).

Table 12. Life experience as a factor in domestic violence

	Abused (%)	Non-abuse (i%)	P
Know anyone who has been hit by her husband?			<0.001
No	535(35.3)	5514(52.4)	
Yes	744(49.0)	2931(27.8)	
Don't know	238(15.7)	2079(19.8)	
Have seen your father hit your mother?			<0.001
No	994(65.5)	8356(79.4)	
Yes	376(24.8)	1235(11.7)	
Not sure	148(9.7)	933(8.9)	
Know your father-in-law hits your mother-in-law?			<0.001
No	566(37.3)	5698(54.1)	
Yes	230(15.2)	629(6.0)	
Not sure	722(47.5)	4196(39.9)	

3.5 Couple's relationship

The results show that the abused women were more likely to have poor relationships with their husbands (p<0.001) (see Table 13).

3.6 Domestic violence and women's reproductive health

The abused women were more likely to have more pregnancies, deliveries, spontaneous abortions and abortions (p<0.05) (see Table 14) than the non-abused.

Table 13. Couple's relationship as a factor in domestic violence

	Abused (%)	Non-abused (%)	P
Are you afraid of your husband?			<0.001
No	1115 (73.5)	9288 (88.3)	
Yes	403 (26.5)	1235 (11.7)	
Do you quarrel with your husband?			<0.001
No or few	208 (13.7)	3448 (32.8)	
Yes	1310 (86.3)	7071 (67.2)	
Does your husband ignore you?			<0.001
No	991 (65.3)	9178 (87.2)	
Yes	527 (34.7)	1346 (12.8)	
Does your husband damage your treasures or pets on purpose?			<0.001
No	1299 (85.6)	10171 (96.7)	
Yes	219 (14.6)	352 (3.3)	
Is your husband angry if you talk with another man?			<0.001
No	924 (60.9)	8709 (82.8)	
Yes	594 (39.1)	1815 (17.2)	
Does he put pressure on you to deliver a boy?			<0.001
No	1214 (80.0)	9897 (94.0)	
Yes	304 (20.0)	627 (6.0)	
Do you get his agreement before going to see a doctor?			<0.001
No	1026 (67.6)	8093 (76.9)	
Yes	492 (32.4)	2431 (23.1)	
Is your husband always reluctant to give you money when you need it?			<0.001
No	1166 (76.8)	9642 (91.6)	
Yes	352 (23.2)	880 (8.4)	

Table 14. Domestic violence and history of pregnancy

	Abused (%)	Non-abused (%)	P
Number of pregnancies			<0.001
1	762 (50.3)	6865 (65.3)	
more then 1	753 (49.7)	3652 (34.7)	
Number of deliveries			<0.05
1	1461 (96.3)	10232 (97.2)	
more then 1	56 (3.7)	293 (2.8)	
Number of spontaneous abortions			
0	1328 (87.5)	9485 (90.2)	
1 or more	190 (12.5)	1034 (9.8)	
Number of abortions			<0.001
0	903 (59.5)	7746 (73.6)	
1 or more	615 (40.5)	2777 (26.4)	

It was also found that an abused woman was more likely to have a history of vaginal bleeding during previous pregnancies and a history of poor obstetric outcome (P<0.05) (see Table 15).

Table 15. DVT and poor obstetric history

	Abused (%)	Non-abused (%)	P
History of vaginal bleeding during previous pregnancy			<0.05
No	1433 (94.4)	10067 (95.7)	
Yes	85 (5.6)	454 (4.3)	
History of poor obstetric outcome			<0.01
No	1413 (93.1)	9984 (94.8)	
Yes	105 (6.9)	542 (5.2)	

Moreover, the abused women were more likely to have started prenatal check-ups late (p<0.01) and have more prenatal check-up visits (P<0.05) (see Table 16).

Table 16. Prenatal check-ups and domestic violence

	Abused (%)	Non-abused (%)	P
The first prenatal check-up at			<0.001
<12 weeks	1098 (72.4)	8191 (77.9)	
12 - 35 weeks	414 (27.3)	2305 (21.9)	
>36 weeks	4 (0.3)	22 (0.2)	
Number of prenatal check-ups			<0.05
<5	176 (11.6)	1473 (14.0)	
5-10	825 (54.4)	5266 (50.0)	
>11	516 (34.0)	3784 (36.0)	

The results of questions on domestic violence and poor obstetric outcome during the latest pregnancy show that an abused woman was more likely to have pregnancy anaemia and other poor obstetric outcomes (p<0.001) (see Table 17).

Table 17. Domestic violence and poor obstetric outcome

	Abused (%)	Non-abused (%)	P
Vaginal bleeding during pregnancy			>0.05
No	1310 (86.3)	9573 (90.9)	
Yes	208 (13.7)	953 (9.1)	
Pregnancy anaemia			<0.001
No	1245 (82.0)	9441 (89.7)	
Yes	273 (18.0)	1085 (10.3)	
Poor obstetric outcome			<0.001
No	1212 (79.8)	9094 (86.4)	
Yes	306 (20.2)	1432 (13.6)	

3.7 Domestic violence and women's psychological status

(a) Postnatal depression

The rate of postnatal depression in the abused women was 31.7% and 19.3% among the non-abused women. Thus the abused women were more likely to suffer from postnatal depression than the non-abused (p<0.001). In addition, the proportion of women with severe depression in the abused group was significantly higher (P<0.01) than in the non-abused group.

Table 18. Severity of depression by abuse

Severity of Depression	Abused (%)	Non-abused (%)
Light	336 (69.9)	1528 (75.2)
Medium	120 (24.9)	448 (22.0)
Severe	25 (5.2)	57 (2.8)

(b) Emotions after delivery

After delivery, women were more likely to be abused if they themselves, their husbands or their parents-in-law were unhappy (p<0.001).

Table 19. Domestic violence and emotions after delivery

After you delivered the baby,	Abused (%)	Non-abused (%)	P
Were you			<0.001
unhappy?	42 (2.8)	124 (1.2)	
neutral?	115 (7.6)	495 (4.7)	
Happy?	1361 (89.7)	9906 (94.1)	
Was your husband			<0.001
unhappy?	25 (1.7)	59 (0.6)	
neutral?	94 (6.3)	306 (2.9)	
happy?	1374 (92.0)	10062 (96.5)	
Were your parents-in-law			<0.001
unhappy?	50 (3.5)	103 (1.0)	
neutral?	113 (8.0)	456 (4.5)	
happy?	1252 (88.5)	9610 (94.5)	

3.8 Babies' health status and domestic violence

(a) Neonates' physical status and domestic violence

Higher neonate morbidity was found in babies of abused women (p<0.001). However, no relationship was found between domestic violence and birth weight (P>0.05) (see Table 20).

Table 20. Neonates' status and domestic violence

	Abused (%)	Non-abused (%)	P
Birth weight			>0.05
<2500g	29 (1.9)	171 (1.6)	
2500~4000g	1393 (91.8)	9799 (93.1)	
>4000g	96 (6.3)	550 (5.2)	
Neonates' illness			<0.001
No	1453 (95.7)	10284 (97.7)	
Yes	65 (4.3)	240 (2.3)	

(b) Domestic violence and babies' behaviour

Among babies aged older than one year, it was found that those of abused women were more likely to have 'attack' behaviour, negative emotions, poor adaptability and withdrawal (p<0.01).

4. Effects of abuse on women's reproductive health

4.1 Effects of domestic violence during pregnancy on maternal complications

Since poor obstetric outcome happens rarely, the study combined various complications into one category for analysis. Poor obstetric outcomes in this instance include preterm delivery, intrauterine growth retardation, fetal death, neonatal death, placental abruption, premature rupture of membranes, first or second trimester bleeding, and anaemia during pregnancy. The results of logistic regression analysis show that factors influencing poor obstetric outcome include domestic violence during pregnancy, a history of spontaneous abortion, abortion, higher education, being a white-collar worker and alcohol use. Women abused during pregnancy were found to be 1.78 times more likely to have poor obstetric outcomes, while women with a history of spontaneous abortion were 1.88 times more likely to have poor obstetric outcomes, and women with a history of assisted abortion were 1.48 times more likely to have poor obstetric outcomes. The incidence of poor obstetric outcome increased by 65% and 76% respectively, when the women had graduated from senior high school or college (see Table 21).

Table 21. Factors influencing poor obstetric outcome

Variable	B	Wald	P	OR	OR95%CI Lower	Upper
Domestic violence during pregnancy	0.58	30.28	0.00	1.78	1.45	2.18
Spontaneous abortion	0.63	69.43	0.00	1.88	1.62	2.19
Assisted abortion	0.39	68.74	0.00	1.48	1.35	1.62
Level of education		30.09	0.00			
Primary						
Junior high	0.21	0.96	0.30	1.23	0.81	1.86
Senior high	0.50	5.79	0.02	1.65	1.10	2.47
College or above	0.56	7.15	0.01	1.76	1.16	2.65
White collar	0.11	4.48	0.03	1.12	1.01	1.24
Use alcohol	0.18	7.16	0.01	1.19	1.05	1.36

4.2 Effects of domestic violence after pregnancy on postnatal depression

The results of logistic regression analysis show domestic violence after pregnancy, types of family, educational level, occupation, income, poor obstetric outcome and neonatal illness as factors related to postnatal depression. Women abused after pregnancy were found to be 1.92 times more likely to have postnatal depression, while women who lived in extended families were 0.91 times less likely, and women who lived alone were 1.93 times more likely. The incidence of postnatal depression decreased to 86%, 74% and 63% respectively, when the women had graduated from junior high school, senior high school or college, compared with women who had graduated from primary school. White-collar workers appear to be less likely to have postnatal depression (OR=0.84). Thus it would seem that higher income can protect women from postnatal depression. Women with poor obstetric outcomes were 1.15 times more likely to have postnatal depression, and those whose baby had neonatal illness were 1.50 times more likely. (See Table 22).

Table 22. Factors related to postnatal depression

Variables	B	Wald	P	OR	OR95%CI Lower	Upper
Domestic violence after pregnancy	0.65	72.99	0.00	1.92	1.65	2.22
Artificial abortion			0.00			
Level of education						
Primary (R)	-0.14	0.72	0.40	0.86	0.62	1.21
Junior high	-0.30	3.17	0.08	0.74	0.53	1.03
Senior high	-0.47	7.10	0.01	0.63	0.45	0.88
College or above	-0.18	8.66	0.00	0.84	0.74	0.94
Poor obstetric outcome	0.14	6.73	0.09	1.15	1.03	1.28
Income after delivery		0.00				
<300 Yuan						
300-800 Yuan	-0.16	8.28	0.00	0.85	0.77	0.95
>800 Yuan	-0.24	12.93	0.00	0.78	0.69	0.90
Type of family		0.00				
Nuclear						
Extended	-0.10	3.92	0.05	0.91	0.83	0.999
Living alone	0.66	7.21	0.01	1.93	1.20	3.13
Neonatal illness	0.41	9.72	0.00	1.50	1.16	1.95

5. Results of in-depth interviews with abused women

5.1 Sociodemographic characteristics of the interviewed abused women

Twelve women identified as having been abused by their intimate partners were interviewed in depth. Their ages ranged from 25 to 37 years. The majority (9/12) had graduated from at least senior high school. Their occupations varied. The majority were unemployed or had been laid off. However, there were also some white-collar female workers (technicians, officers, nurses) among the interviewed survivors of domestic violence. One-third (8/12) of those interviewed had no income, and the incomes of the others were also not high. Almost all the abused women were in their first marriage, except one for whom it was her second marriage.

Comparing the sociodemographic characteristics of the abused women and their partners, it was found that, in all but two cases, the abused women were younger than their partners. For most of the couples (8/12) the educational level of both partners was the same. There were three cases where an abused woman's level of education was lower than that of her partner. However, there was only one case where the woman's educational level was higher than that of her husband. More abused women were employed than their husbands. In half of the couples, the woman's income was lower than that of her husband.

In summary, most of the abused women were younger than their partners. There was no relationship between the women's educational level and maltreatment. Many educated women were suffering from domestic violence. There was also no relationship between the partner's educational level and battering. Most of the abused women were more socioeconomically disadvantaged than their partners.

Table 23. Sociodemographic characteristics of abused women and their partners

	Abused women	Partners
Age (years old)	25-37	26-45
Educational level		
Junior high school	3	3
Senior high school	5	4
University	4	5
Occupation		
Unemployed, laid off	7	4
Worker	2	4
Technician, officer, nurse	3	4
Income (Yuan/per month)		
No income	3	0
<=1000	9	11
>1000	0	1
Marital statue		
First marriage	11	10
Remarriage	1	2

5.2 Domestic violence situation

Among the 12 battered women interviewed, six were abused during pregnancy but the abuse was not limited to that period. Since the women interviewed were those who had babies between 6 and 18 months of age, most of them had married within the previous five years. Despite the short period of marriage, abuse for many had happened repeatedly before, during and after pregnancy. One woman, married for three years, started being abused two months after her marriage, and the abuse continued. However, all the women who had been abused prior to becoming pregnant said that their husbands' battering decreased during pregnancy.

Physical abuse is usually accompanied by sexual and psychological abuse. The most severe reported case of physical abuse was bruising. However, most of the survivors in the study were not beaten at the most severe end of the physical-abuse scale. Most women mentioned that cursing often happened. If the cursing became severe, battering often followed. One woman reported:

> *At the time I was sitting on the bed and holding my son. He threw a bowl of milk at me on the seventh day after delivery. I didn't say anything. After that, I cleaned the floor and the bed. Suddenly, he jumped on me and beat me seriously.*

The violence could take forms other than physical abuse. In some cases, there was emotional abuse. The women thought that this was much worse than physical pain. One woman described her husband's emotional abuse in these terms:

> *He took off my clothes, threw them on the ground, trampled on them and urinated on them. It was painful in the depth of my heart.*

Many women said that they had a "cold war" frequently, which was always followed by abuse or quarrelling. Sometimes such cold wars lasted for months with no communication whatsoever. One woman claimed:

> *It is so normal for us to have cold wars for two months.*

> *We didn't talk to each other for three weeks after I was abused. One day, my daughter got a fever and I asked him to take her to hospital. From that day on, we started talking to each other.*

Such long periods of silence are harmful to the mental health of both the woman and her partner. The biochemical changes in women during pregnancy and after giving birth result in mood swings. Those physiological aspects are exacerbated by social difficulties in adjusting to the transition to motherhood and the resulting stress. Women often become preoccupied with their babies and the increased household work after delivery and are less able, physically and emotionally, to tend to their husbands' needs. In the study population, many women reported that such factors could lead to frequent sexual abuse.

5.3 Reasons for wife battering

Some women thought that they were battered, not because they were doing anything wrong, but because of the hot-tempered, irrational behaviour of their husbands. So they forgave them. One interviewee reported:

> While we were discussing, he didn't agree with me. Then he battered me. I have no choice. His personality is like that –easily irritated and hot tempered. I have to suffer since it is impossible to change his personality.

The most frequently reported reasons for battering women were: disharmonious relationships with in-laws, financial conflicts, alcohol consumption by the husband, household chore issues, and extramarital relationships of the husband.

The traditional concepts guiding the division of labour within the family, as well as the standards of behaviour, are still widely accepted by older Chinese people. However, the new generation is educated and often both partners in a marriage are engaged in outside work. The gap between the two generations can make for a disharmonious in-law relationship. The women interviewed said that their parents-in-law believed that a daughter-in-law was responsible for taking care of the whole family. Therefore, after work, the daughter-in-law should cook, wash for them and clean the house, although the parents-in-law may not be old, and may stay at home the whole day. The women were dissatisfied with that situation. When that type of conflict erupted, the son would usually take the side of his parents. For example, one woman explained:

> Whenever my mother-in-law visits and stays at my house, we have a quarrel and I am battered. My mother-in-law is less than sixty years old. She stays at home the whole day with nothing to do. But I have to work the whole day. After going back home, I felt tired and had a rest for about one hour. After that I started cooking. So my mother-in-law was angry with me and complained that the dinner was too late and so on.

> Mother-in-law only needs to say a few vague words like 'she and I had a quarrel earlier today', which will make me be beaten.

Although, women earn money, men always try to control the family's finances and often financial management is a source of abusive behaviour. As one women said:

> I lent our money to his good friend, and his friend promised to return it soon. Since I didn't ask his permission, it caused his battering. In fact, it is his friend, not mine.

However, economic reasons or family conflict are not sufficient to explain abuse. As Heise's ecological model for the explanation of domestic violence stresses, a variety of distal and proximal factors operate in any instance of intimate partner abuse[68]. One factor which pervades both distal and proximate factors is male power. For example, one woman who was interviewed explained how her husband displayed his power over her.

> I didn't know how to please him. I was beaten in every case. For example, when I served him tea, I didn't cover it completely. It caused a beating.

> Every time he is drunk, he beats me.

---

[68] Heise, L. Violence against women: an integrated ecological framework. *Violence Against Women*, 1998, 4, 262-290

Two women had been battered when they found out their husbands were having extramarital affairs. The women had wanted to stop them. One woman described her husband's response to being found out:

> *One day at 23:00, my husband had not come back home. Therefore, I went out to look for him. Finally, I saw him walking with a woman hand-in-hand and I followed him. When he discovered me, he cursed me and battered me. He forced me to accept the fact that he had a lover.*

Such examples illustrate how men enforce their power: they establish their authority by battering their wives.

Four women said that their husbands did not like them to take care of their own families. Frequently, after they returned from their parents' house, their husbands would curse and batter them. It was their husbands' view that a wife should relinquish responsibility for her own family and concentrate on caring for her husband's family.

Another factor identified by the women as leading to violence was a wife complaining that her husband did not do the household chores. After a birth, household chores increase, but husbands do not help their wives to relieve the burden of household tasks. One woman explained the dual burden of paid work and housework and the effect it had on her and her relationship with her husband, culminating in abuse.

> *My husband always said his work was too busy to come back early. During the first month that I started work after the birth, I nearly went crazy. I am a nurse director. So I am busy during working hours. After work, I was very tired. However, I had to do the cooking, washing and cleaning - everything. He did not help me at all. (My housemaid only stayed at my house during the daytime). I felt very bad. So we always quarreled and several times he battered me as I babbled.*

5.4. Women's actions after abuse

It was observed that some of the abused women had a fairly strong awareness of gender equality, although the results of the gender role awareness test suggested that, on the whole, women in the larger survey had serious gaps in their understanding of gender roles. Some of the women were sensitive to male chauvinism and discrimination against women, but did not feel that they had the strength or power to retaliate effectively. When suffering from beating, the battered women behaved in various ways, from cursing back (8) to hitting back (8). The women said that, although they hit back, they suffered much more than men.

> *Men's beating gives us pain, not like us. We are weak and cannot make them feel pain.*

However, one woman said,

> *I don't do anything. Just let him beat me. One time he battered me and I hit back. After that he battered me more seriously.*

Concealment and acceptance were the main reactions reported by most women when beaten for the first time. They even concealed the beating from their families, who were the closest and most sympathetic when they were miserable. The question that must be raised here is: why do they keep silent? Do they quickly forget or forgive their husbands' violent actions after being beaten? The answer is no. The possible reasons are that they think that their families cannot do anything besides worry. As one women said,

> *If I told my parents I was battered, they would worry about me. Therefore, whenever I go to my parent's house, I have to pretend nothing has happened between us.*

Women also do not tell others. They reported feeling ashamed to tell others about their misery since they could not escape from public **perceptions and opinions, which assume that "there is no smoke without fire".**

> *If people knew about my husband's bad actions, I would be the person who felt shameful and would 'lose face'. They might also think I am a bad woman.*
>
> *It is a private matter. If outsiders had known my situation, they would have laughed at me. I would have lost face and couldn't have dared to meet others.*

The ridicule and comments of neighbours can make it difficult to live a normal life. The reputation of the family is the highest priority for many women. Personal grievances are seen as unimportant in the bigger scheme of things. To earn their neighbours' high regard, women must pretend they are enjoying a happy family life. There is also the issue of self-esteem and standing within the community.

However, if the situation is too severe to solve alone, the first choice is to ask relatives, such as in-laws or parents, or good friends for help. Usually the abused woman will tell her relatives and friends what happened, listen to their opinions and ask them to persuade the violator to behave differently. People believe that "if the family lives in harmony, all will be prosperous." Therefore, friends always try to persuade an abused woman to endure her suffering, even although they may sympathize with her and want to help her.

> *When my husband beat me, I went to my parents-in-law or my family to seek help from them.*
>
> *I did not go to my parents' house. I did not want my parents to know I had been beaten. Therefore, I always went to my husband's friend's house, seeking help from him.*
>
> *I went to the house of my husband's good friend to ask him to persuade my husband not treat me like that.*
>
> *I never went to my neighbour's house. It is useless and would maybe make things worse. In fact, while I was being beaten, a neighbour came. My husband beat me more seriously since he wanted to show his power.*

Several women also said that, if a family member or friends could not solve the violence problem, they did not know where else to seek help.

5.5 Effectiveness of seeking help from society

Three women thought the support they received was effective and four thought it was effective temporarily. Two women felt they failed to get what they needed.

Obviously, there are few social support services for battered women. The public pays little attention to the victims of domestic violence. Instead, wife abuse is regarded as a private affair. Thus battered women often refuse to seek social support and in many cases, even if they do seek services outside the home, such services do not exist.

5.6 Impacts on women and children

Several women thought their lives were not too bad. Although they were beaten, they were generally satisfied with their lives.

> *My friends always admire me for having a good husband, since my husband does many household chores. He looks after my son, does cooking and washing. He does these thing better than me. He is a good husband if he is not beating me. But his personality is that way. I forgive him.*

Thus doing household chores makes a good husband in the eyes of the some abused women, family members, outsiders and public opinion generally.

However, abuse causes many women to become depressed and anxious. They do not like to tell people for fear of ridicule, and endure the harm silently, which makes them more depressed. From their point of view, talking to people around them does not help their plight.

When the researchers met the interviewees, the abused women were very talkative. They revealed a lot about their personal lives and did not seem to be concealing anything. That may have been because of their relative anonymity, given that they knew the interviewer was from Beijing rather than from their own community. They appeared to trust the interviewer and did not fear that their neighbours would find out about their situation. After the interview, many women thanked the interviewer many times, saying such things as:

> *I never had a chance like this to talk with someone from deep in my heart. I am very happy today and gained a lot from you. What I want is please don't tell my story to anyone in my community.*

The researchers promised never to reveal details that would identify the interviewees and this was reinforced in the plain language statement given to the interviewees as part of the ethical procedures to gain their consent to participate in the study.

Besides the psychological effects, several of the women had suffered pelvic infections, back pain, headaches and other ailments associated with stress. They also worried about their children's educational issues and thought that their situation was not good for their children's development.

Many studies show that wife abuse is often accompanied by child abuse, and abusive husbands are likely to be abusive fathers. However, in this study, only three abusive husbands were reported to also beat their children. The others were said to treat their children well.

> *He loves my daughter and never beats her.*

> *He is very patient with my son. He would like to take care of my son, prepare his meals etc. He treats my son better than me.*

It seems that abusive men have double standards. Possibly, having only one child in the family increases the value of children, as people often call the child a "little emperor".

As for the three abusive husbands who beat their children, one was remarried. He had a daughter aged 15 years. He did not want the second child when his wife conceived. He wanted his wife to have an abortion, but his wife insisted on keeping the baby.

> *I couldn't leave my son alone with him. I was afraid my husband would treat him badly or beat him. When my son cried, he always shouted at him and sometimes beat him.*

The other two, although they had only one child, still beat their children.

5.7 Marriages of abused women

After abuse, two couples' relationships went back to normal. Six women had no thoughts of divorce or departure. Three women were hesitant about divorce and one was going through divorce proceedings.

> *My husband is very handsome. I love him very much. Even if he beats me and he sleeps with other women, I love him. I hope he can change his behaviour later. I don't want to leave him.*

In summary, the in-depth interviews revealed violence against pregnant women before, during and after pregnancy. All three types of violence (physical, psychological and sexual) are going on and some cases are severe and persistent. Many educated women suffer from domestic violence. There appears to be no relationship between the partner's educational level and battering, but most of the abused women were more disadvantaged socioeconomically than their partners. Society and the public in the research areas regard domestic violence as a private issue. Although women might be strong in some cases, ultimately they feel they do not have the power to fight back or stop their husbands' behaviour. They often try to resist domestic violence, but the social network to support abused women is very weak and many are too afraid to shame their families by revealing the extent of their abuse to anyone.

CONCLUSIONS

As far as the writers are aware, this is the first community-based study in China to examine women's postpartum experience of domestic violence in addition to abuse before and during pregnancy. Although the results of the study cannot be generalized for all of China, the major findings do provide representative information regarding domestic violence against women before, during, and after pregnancy in northern China.

1. Prevalence of domestic violence

According to the study, the prevalence rate of domestic violence occurring in any period before, during or after pregnancy was 12.6%, which is consistent with other studies where the prevalence rates of domestic violence ranged from 9.7% to 29.7% [69,70,71,72,73,74]. However, the actual prevalence rate may be higher than the results suggest, given the traditional belief that domestic 'shame' should not be made public, and the fact that some women only count severe abuse as violence. It is important to note that, given the large population in the areas of China covered by the study, even the reported prevalence translates into a huge number of abused women.

The prevalence of domestic violence during the approximately nine months of pregnancy (4.3%) was relatively low compared with prevalence during the 12 months before pregnancy (9.1%) and after delivery (8.3%) during the mean 11 months postpartum period studied. The figures are similar to those found by a 1999 study of American Chinese, where the prevalence of abuse during a current pregnancy was 4.3%[75]. Although reports correlating abuse and pregnancy have emphasized the potential for increased abuse during pregnancy[76,77,78,79], several studies support the findings of this study[80,81]. The findings are consistent with the qualitative study, where women reported that abuse had decreased rather than increased with pregnancy.

Many studies show that wife abuse is often accompanied by child abuse, and abusive husbands are likely to be abusive fathers. However, the qualitative study found that, unlike other country studies but similar to the study of Chinese by Meng[82], more abusive husbands did not beat their children. Presumably, the one-child policy in China increases the value of children. The fewer children one has, the more precious each child becomes. Therefore, the lower prevalence of domestic violence during pregnancy might result from the short period of the study and/or the value placed on the child in the context of the one-child policy.

For many of the women in the study, physical abuse was not an isolated event but an ongoing phenomenon, often accompanied by debilitating sexual and psychological abuse. Results show a strong association between physical, sexual and psychological abuse, with nearly one-third of the women

---

[69] Helton A, Mcfarlane J, Anderson ET. Battered and pregnant: A prevalence study. *American Journal of Public Health*, 1987, 77:1337-1339.
[70] *Op cit.* Ref 17.
[71] Gazamararian JA *et al.* The relationship between pregnancy intendedness and physical violence during pregnancy. *Obstetrics and Gynecology*, 1995, 85:1031-1038
[72] *Op cit.* Ref 3.
[73] *Op cit.* Ref 1.
[74] *Op cit.* Ref. 2.
[75] Leung WC *et al.* The prevalence of domestic violence against pregnant women in a Chinese community. *International Journal of Gynaecology and Obstetrics*, 1999 Jul, 66(1): 23-30.
[76] Stark E, Flitcraft A, Frazier W. Medicine and patriarchal violence: The social construction of a "private" event. *International Journal of Health Services*, 1979, 9:461.
[77] Purwar MB *et al.* Survey of physical abuse during pregnancy GMCH, Nagpur, India. *Journal of Obstetrical and Gynaecological Research*, 1999 Jun, 25(3): 165-171.
[78] *Op cit.* Ref 17.
[79] Martin SL *et al.* Physical abuse of women before, during, and after pregnancy *Journal of the American Medical Association*, 2001, 285:1581-1583.
[80] *Op cit.* Ref 75.
[81] *Op cit.* Ref 2.
[82] Meng L, Cecilia C. Enduring violence and staying in marriage. *Violence against Women*, 1999, 5:1469-1492.

experiencing more than one type of domestic violence, which is consistent with the findings of other studies[83,84]. For example, research suggests that physical violence in intimate relationships is always accompanied by psychological abuse, and in one-third to over one-half of cases by sexual violence[85].

Many of the women who suffered any domestic violence generally experienced multiple acts over time; half of them were abused more than once. That finding is consistent with other studies such as that of Ellsberg, in which 60% of women were abused more than once in the year prior to the study[86].

In terms of severity, most instances of violence were not perceived by the women interviewed as being at the severe end of the violence scale, which is different from Dr. Peicheng's study in 1996[87]. However, it must be remembered that Peicheng's study was conducted in the psychology clinic of a hospital, where patients had severe psychological problems and were thus more likely to have been exposed to severe violence. The current study is a community-based study, which reflects the general population more accurately. Since domestic violence occurs in the family and most instances are not perceived by the women as severe, it is generally ignored by the women, their families and broader society.

Analysis of the results by province shows that there is an inverse relationship between level of economic and social development and prevalence of domestic violence. That relationship even overrides the rural/urban difference in domestic violence levels, with prevalence being high even in large cities in the least developed provinces. In developing prevention strategies, attention should be paid to that clear relationship.

2. Pattern of domestic violence before, during and after pregnancy

Two of the most important findings of the study are that domestic violence before pregnancy is a strong risk factor for domestic violence during and after pregnancy, and that domestic violence during a previous period is a strong risk factor for subsequent domestic violence, a finding consistent with other research documenting the often long-term nature of violence[88,89]. Those findings should alert health care providers to the fact that women who are abused before and/or during pregnancy often continue to experience abuse after infant delivery, placing the health of both mother and child in jeopardy. Routine screening for domestic violence in maternity service settings is therefore advocated as a means of decreasing the effects on women and their unborn children.

3. Women's actions in response to domestic violence

The qualitative results from the interviews confirm the quantitative findings that most abused women are not passive victims but hit back and use active strategies to maximize their safety. Some women resist, others flee, and still others attempt to keep the peace by capitulating to their husbands' demands. In terms of seeking help, the most common action is to not talk to anyone initially. However, if the violence is too severe to endure, the women will seek help first from family members.

A woman's response to abuse is often limited by the options available to her. Fear of retribution, lack of alternative means of economic support, concern for her children, emotional dependence, lack of support from family and friends, and an abiding hope that "he will change" are common factors that keep women in abusive relationships. At the same time, fear of social stigma often prevents women from reaching out for help. Moreover, it is clear that those who do reach out do so primarily to family members and friends, rather than formal institutions. Therefore, it is necessary to equip family members and

---

[83] Ellsberg MC *et al*. Wife abuse among women of childbearing age in Nicaragua. *American Journal of Public Health*, 1999, 89:241-244.
[84] Yoshihama M, Sorenson SB. Physical, and sexual and emotional abuse by male intimates: experiences of women in Japan. *Violence and Victims*, 1994, 9:63-77.
[85] *Ibid*.
[86] *Op cit*. Ref 83.
[87] Peicheng H. Survey on domestic violence in 200 couples. *China Psychological Health*, 1996, 10(4): 171-2
[88] *Op cit*. Ref 79.
[89] *Op cit*. Ref 69.

friends so that they can help abused women effectively. At the same time, however, action should be taken in the formal sector (e.g. police, law) and NGOs to help abused women actively and effectively.

4. Women's attitudes towards domestic violence and gender roles

Only one-fifth of the women surveyed did not agree that "family problems should only be discussed with family members", and only one-tenth agreed that "if a man mistreats his wife, others outside the family should intervene". Therefore, many women perceive domestic violence as a private affair, which limits an abused woman's motivation to seek outside help.

In terms of gender roles, most of the women were not clear about gender roles and rights. In the last decade in northern China, more and more women have been educated at the tertiary level and have become professionals. They live in a period of social transition, where they have many opportunities but are still restricted by the persistence of traditional beliefs and values. On the one hand, they have knowledge about gender equality; on the other, they are also influenced by traditional family concepts. Therefore, women are not sure about their roles and their rights. There is an urgent need to educate both men and women on gender roles in all situations, including at the community level.

5. Possible factors associated with domestic violence

5.1 Lower socioeconomic status

The study results show that, compared with their husbands, the abused women were in lower socioeconomic status groups in terms of education, occupation and income. Women's socioeconomic status worsens after delivery. Bivariate analysis shows that one predictor of higher rates of abuse is lower socioeconomic status in both women and their spouses. The study results thus support the findings that, although domestic violence cuts across all socioeconomic groups, women living in poverty are disproportionately more affected[90,91,92,93,94,95]. Although equal status in the family and in society has been advocated in China for many years, in general, women's status is still lower than that of their spouses, thus maintaining a system whereby women depend on their husbands and suffer and endure abuse perceiving that they have no alternative.

Traditionally, men in China have taken total responsibility for the economic and social standing of the family. When a man's socioeconomic status is low, his capacity to perform that traditional role is undermined. Quarrels often result because a man feels compromised in his capacity as the primary breadwinner, and battering his wife to re-assert his authority in the family can be a consequence. Empowerment of women is therefore essential in preventing domestic violence. However, men also need to find other avenues to empowerment than violence. A multisectoral approach to the problem is needed, whereby policies and services address the sequalae of low socioeconomic status in terms of gender roles for both men and women.

5.2 Living in an extended family or living alone

The abused women were found to be more likely to live in an extended family or live alone, which is consistent with other studies[96,97]. Living alone may be the result of domestic violence. However, it is easier for family conflict to develop in an extended family living arrangement. Therefore, more abuse was found in that group.

---

[90] Dearwater SR et al. Prevalence of intimate partner abuse in women treated at community hospital emergency departments. *Journal of the American Medical Association*, 1998, 280:433-438.
[91] Hathaway JE et al. Health status and health care use of Massachusetts women reporting partner abuse. *American Journal of Preventive Medicine*, 2000, 19: 302-307.
[92] Coker AL et al. Frequency and correlates of intimate partner violence by type: physical, sexual, and psychological battering. *American Journal of Public Health*, 2000, 90: 553-539.
[93] Grimstad H et al. Physical abuse and low birth weight: a case –control study. *British Journal of Obstetrics and Gynaecology*, 1997 Nov, 104(11): 1281-1287.
[94] Martin SL et al. Domestic Violence in northern India. *American Journal of Epidemiology*, 1999, 150:417-26.
[95] *Op cit.* Ref 83.
[96] *Op cit.* Ref. 69
[97] *Op cit.* Ref 77.

5.3 Substance abuse

The abused women and their spouses were significantly more likely to smoke and use alcohol, which is similar to the findings of earlier studies[98][99][100]. Perpetrators were also found to be more likely to be illicit drug users. Therefore, prevention of domestic violence should also focus on substance use and abuse.

5.4 Gender roles and women's rights awareness

The result shows that the higher the gender role awareness, the lower the rate of domestic violence. Therefore, it is necessary to encourage training of both women and men on gender roles and women's rights.

5.5 Poor relationship between couples

The positive associations between fear of partner, quarrels between couples and domestic violence, which was similarly found in Purwar's 1999 study[101], suggest that a woman reporting fear of her partner or quarrels may be a strong indicator of domestic violence. Marriage mediation should be undertaken at the early stage of quarrelling to prevent domestic violence.

5.6 Experience of domestic violence

Another risk factor that appeared was being a witness to domestic violence, which is consistent with other studies[102]. Findings confirm that domestic violence is learnt behavior. Women witnessing domestic violence are more likely to experience domestic violence, while men who witness domestic violence are more likely to become perpetrators of that violence.

5.7 Poor obstetric history

Women who live with violent partners have a difficult time protecting themselves from unwanted pregnancy. Violence can lead directly to unwanted pregnancy, or indirectly by interfering with the woman's ability to use contraceptives. The study found that abused women were significantly more likely to have a poor obstetric history e.g. more pregnancies, abortions and other poor obstetric outcomes, which is similar to the findings of other studies[103,104,105,106,107].

5.8 Late prenatal check-up

Abused pregnant women tend to start prenatal check-ups during their second or third trimester, which is later than non-abused women. That prevents early detection of problems, which may have direct or indirect effects on the growing fetus[108][109]. However, the study also found that, once they start to attend prenatal clinics, abused women tend to have more prenatal check-ups than non-abused women. Such a pattern of prenatal clinic usage may reflect the abusive partner initially preventing his wife from attending prenatal check-ups but, once she has finally started, she attends frequently since she worries about the welfare of the unborn child.

---

[98] *Op cit.* Ref 17.
[99] *Op cit.* Ref 77.
[100] Fernandez FM, Krueger PM. Domestic violence: Effect on pregnancy outcome. *Journal of the American Osteopath Association*, 1999 May, 99(5): 254-256.
[101] *Op cit.* Ref 77.
[102] *Op cit.* Ref 1.
[103] *Op cit.* Ref 42.
[104] *Op cit.* Ref 20.
[105] Berenson AB et al. Perinatal morbidity associated with violence experienced by pregnant women. *American Journal of Obstetrics and Gynecology*, 1994, 170:1760-1769.
[106] *Op cit.* Ref 1.
[107] *Op cit.* Ref 2.
[108] Gazmararian JA et al. Prevalence of violence against pregnant women. *Journal of the American Medical Association*, 1996, 275:1915-1920.
[109] *Op cit.* Ref 77.

6. Effects of domestic violence on reproductive health

6.1 The findings on the latest pregnancy of the women interviewed show that poor obstetric outcomes are strongly related to domestic violence during pregnancy. Women abused during pregnancy are at significantly greater risk for poor obstetric outcomes. However, further study is needed, since the obstetric outcome data were collected from the women, but not from the obstetric clinic.

6.2 Effects of domestic violence after pregnancy on postnatal depression. The research found a strong link between postnatal depression and domestic violence after pregnancy. Helton's 1987 study had the same finding[110]

It is obvious from the study that domestic violence has adverse effects on both obstetric outcomes and women's mental health. The study further suggests that abuse should be considered a factor in poor obstetric outcome. Because women with a history of abuse are more likely to tolerate abuse in future relationships, it is possible that prior abuse is a factor in their poor obstetric histories, which in turn increases their conventional biomedical risk. In other words, biomedical risk may actually serve as a proxy for social risk (e.g. abuse). Routine screening in maternity services is strongly advocated.

Chapter 5.
DOMESTIC VIOLENCE AMONG WOMEN SEEKING ABORTIONS

This chapter comprises two parts. In the first part, which presents results of the study, there are three sections: (1) the general characteristics of the 1215 women seeking abortions and their partners; (2) the domestic violence situation among the respondents; and (3) the possible factors related to domestic violence. The second part of the chapter discusses the results.

RESULTS

1. Respondents' characteristics

1.1 Sociodemographic characteristics of respondents and their intimate partners

The sample for this study consisted of 1215 women seeking pregnancy termination in seven northern cities of China.

(a) Age

The average age of the respondents was 27.4 (S.D. 5.6 years) years and their ages ranged from 17 to 46 years. The average age of the women's intimate partners (husbands / boyfriends) was 29.8 (S.D. 5.9 years) and their ages ranged from 18 to 53 years. Nearly one-fifth (19.2%) of the respondents were the same age as their partners. However, most (76.0%) of the respondents were younger than their partners (see Figure 5).

---
[110] *Op cit.* ref 69.

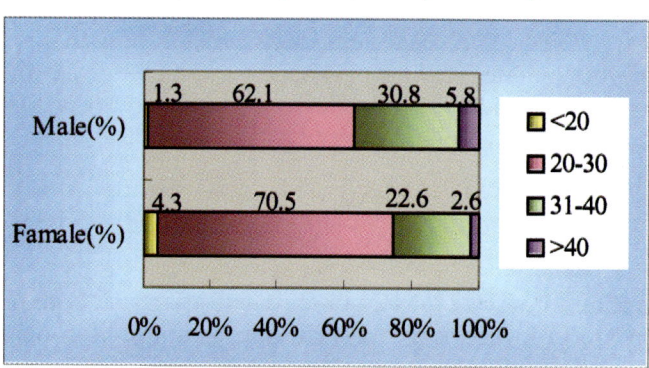

Figure 5. Respondents' and partners' ages

(b) Education

The mean years of education completed by the respondents and their partners were 12.1 (S.D. 2.8 years) and 12.5 (S.D. 2.9 years), respectively. The proportion of respondents and their partners with a higher level of education (senior high school and above) was almost the same (78% vs.80.9%). The difference in years of education between respondents and their partners averaged 0.40 (S.D. 2 years). More than half (55%) of the respondents and their partners had received the same level of education, and 29.3% of the women had educational levels that were lower than those of their partners (see Figure 6).

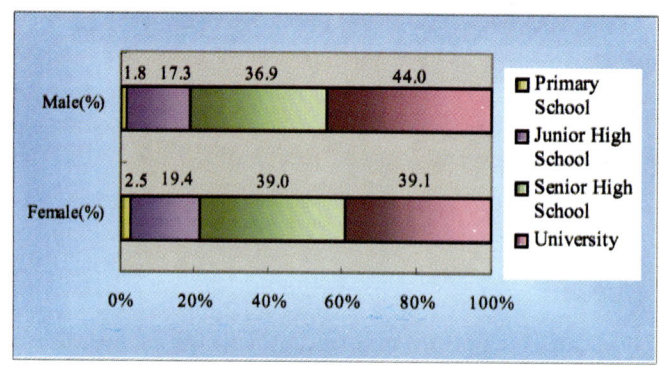

Figure 6. Respondents' and partners' levels of education

(c) Occupation and monthly personal income

The proportion of white-collar workers (including office workers, clerks, professionals, students) among the partners was a little higher than among the respondents (44.7% vs 42.0%). Regarding personal income, 22.8% of the respondents and 6.9% of their partners had monthly personal incomes of less than 300 Yuan, and 50.6% of the partners had monthly incomes of over 800 Yuan, higher than those of the respondents (see Figure 7).

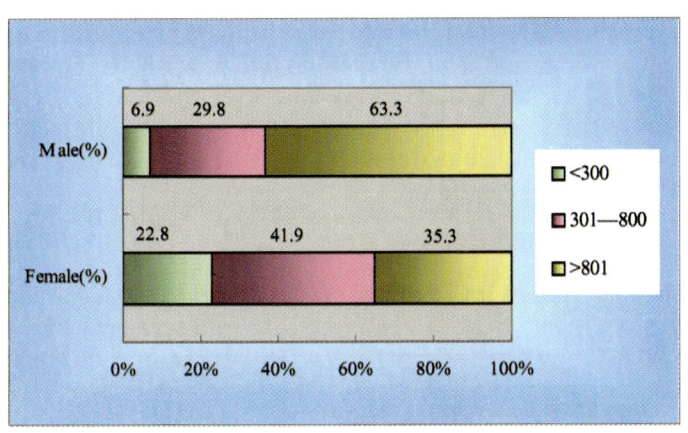

Figure 7. Respondents' and partners' monthly incomes

(d) Marriage

Of the 1215 women studied, 1016 (75.4%) were in their first marriage, 267 (22.8%) were single, 16 (1.3%) were remarried and 6 (0.3%) were divorced. The average length of marriage was 4.9 years; the longest marriage was 24 years. More than one-third (37.3%) of the single and divorced women had known their boyfriends for less than 12 months and 45.3% had lived with their boyfriends.

(5) Personal habits

It was found that 8.6% of the women and 73.7% of their partners smoked, 22.5% of the women and 77.5% of their partners drank alcohol, and 1.3% of the women and 1.8% of their partners abused illegal drugs.

In short, compared with their partners, respondents were younger, had a lower level of education and a lower monthly personal income. Also, most of the respondents were in their first marriage. Very few of the respondents smoked, drank alcohol or used illegal drugs.

1.2 History of abortion and relevant factors

More than half (57.0%) of the women had experienced a previous pregnancy termination, with a mean number of abortions per woman of 0.94. Of those women, 6.7% had experienced spontaneous abortions. The major reason given for the current pregnancy (58%) was non-use of contraception.

Most (94.9%) of the women had undergone their current pregnancy termination after discussing it with their partners. Only 3% had not discussed the termination with their partners. Most women (79.2%) had been willing to have an abortion, but some (2.1%) had undergone the termination because they were compelled to do so by their partners.

The first three leading reasons given for pregnancy termination were "already have a child", "unmarried" and "untimely".

1.3 Women's physical and mental health

Among the 1215 women, the prevalence rate of upper reproductive tract infection was 5.3% and of lower reproductive tract infection 23.1%. Also, 12.8% were of the women were anaemic.

The Self-rating Depression Scale was used to evaluate the women's depression. The results show a 38.3% prevalence of depression, including 24.6% light, 11.6% medium and 2.5% severe depression.

1.4 Relationships with husbands or boyfriends

Regarding the relationships between the women and their husbands or boyfriends, the study revealed that more than half (62.2%) of the women had quarreled with their partners, but only 4% quarreled often; 43.1% reported that their partners would be angry if they talked with other men; 26.2% felt their partners were ignorant or indifferent; 14.6% were afraid of their partners, and 8.5% of them often felt afraid; and about 15% felt that their partners were always unwilling to give them money when they needed it.

1.5 Lifetime experience of domestic violence

One-fifth (19.5%) of the women had witnessed parental violence (father beat mother) when they were children; more than half (52.5%) knew of domestic violence against wives/girlfriends around them; and 7.1% knew that their partners' fathers had abused their wives.

1.6 Attitude toward domestic violence and women's rights

As Table 24 shows, most of the women were positively against domestic violence and had a strong awareness of women's rights.

Table 24. Attitude towards domestic violence and women's rights

Items	Agree	Disagree	Uncertain
1. A good wife should obey her husband even if she disagrees with his thoughts or actions.	96 (7.9)	965 (79.4)	154 (12.7)
2. Family problems should only be discussed with family members.	423 (34.8)	520 (42.8)	174 (14.3)
3. A man should show his wife/partner that he is the head of the family.	267 (22.0)	815 (67.0)	133 (10.9)
4. A woman should be able to choose her own friends, even if her husband disapproves	878 (72.3)	181 (14.9)	155 (12.8)
5. A man has a rational reason to hit his wife, when:			
(a) she does not complete her housekeeping to his satisfaction;	29 (2.4)	1162 (95.6)	24 (2.0)
(b) she disobeys him;	27 (2.2)	1162 (95.6)	26 (2.1)
(c) she refuses to have sexual intercourse with him;	23 (1.9)	1162 (95.6)	30 (2.5)
(d) she asks him whether he has other girlfriends; or	35 (2.8)	1129 (92.9)	50 (4.1)
(e) he suspects that she is unfaithful.	112 (9.2)	1008 (83.0)	95 (7.8)

2. Domestic violence among women seeking abortions

2.1 Prevalence of domestic violence in different periods

As shown in Table 25, 274 (22.6%) of the women seeking abortions reported a history of domestic violence (including emotional, sexual and physical abuse). Of the abused women, 220 (18.1%) reported that they had been exposed to sexual violence only, 92 (7.8%) to physical violence only, and 37 (3.0%) to emotional violence only.

Table 25 and Figure 5 also show the prevalence of different types of domestic violence before and after the current pregnancy. The prevalence rate of domestic violence before pregnancy was 21.7%, but it dropped to 7.0% after pregnancy.

In addition, as shown in Figure 6, 21.7% of the women had experienced domestic violence only, but 28.4% of them had suffered domestic violence continually during the current pregnancy. In addition, 10 women had only started to be exposed to domestic violence during their current pregnancy.

Table 25. Prevalence of different types of domestic violence during different periods among women seeking abortions

Period	Domestic violence (N=274) N (%)		Psychological abuse (N=37) N (%)		Sexual abuse (N=220) N (%)		Physical abuse (N=92) N (%)	
Before pregnancy	264	(21.7)	34	(2.8)	210	(17.3)	91	(7.5)
After pregnancy	85	(7.0)	16	(1.3)	60	(4.9)	22	(1.8)
Total	274	(22.6)	37	(3)	220	(18.1)	92	(7.8)

2.2 Times and types of domestic violence

As shown in Table 26, most of the abused women had suffered from domestic violence fewer than 10 times, and 40.5% of them had been exposed to domestic violence only once or twice. A much smaller proportion of the women had been exposed to domestic violence throughout their lives.

The most common type of domestic violence was sexual abuse. Nearly two-thirds (59.5%) of the women had suffered from sexual abuse only. The next most common category was physical abuse (16.1%), followed by emotional abuse only (1.4%). Of the abused women, 77.0% had suffered from one type of abuse only, 18.6% from two types, and 4.4% of them had experienced three types of abuse. Sexual abuse was often followed by physical abuse. The percentages of different types of domestic violence reported are shown in Figure 8.

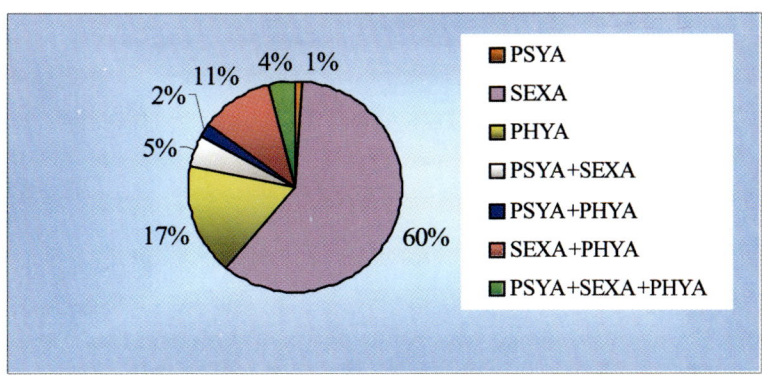

Figure 8. Different types of domestic violence against women seeking abortions, percentages

Table 26. Number of times and types of domestic violence among women seeking abortions

Number of times	Domestic violence (N=274) N (%)		Sexual abuse (N=220) N (%)		Emotional abuse (N=37) N (%)		Physical abuse (N=92) N (%)	
1-2	111	(40.5)	100	(45.5)	13	(35.1)	52	(56.5)
3-10	117	(42.7)	93	(42.3)	13	(35.1)	31	(33.7)
> 10	46	(16.8)	27	(12.2)	11	(29.8)	9	(7.8)

The results also show that 6.3% of the women reported that their partners had required them to indulge in certain sexual activities (oral sex or anal sex) against their will. The proportion was higher in the abused group than the non-abused (15.3% vs 3.6%) (p<0.001).

2.3 Severity of domestic violence

The severity of domestic violence (including emotional, sexual and physical abuse), as reported by the women, is shown in Table 27. Regarding emotional abuse, the most common manner (89.2%) was partners insulting women with dirty words or making them feel bad, while 89.5% of the women who had suffered sexual abuse reported that their partners continuously insisted on having sexual intercourse when they themselves were unwilling. In terms of physical abuse, most (93.5%) of the women who had suffered from physical abuse reported that they had been beaten or pushed, but without causing trauma or persistent pain or limited movement.

Table 27. Severity of domestic violence, by type

Various types and degree of severity	Abused cases	(%)
PSYA (n=37)		
Often insulted you or made you feel bad	33	89.2
Often humiliated you in front of other people	9	24.3
Threatened to divorce or leave you	16	43.2
Threatened to hit you or someone else you care about	7	18.9
Took something with intent to hit you or scare you	10	27.0
SEXA (n=220)		
Continuously insisted you have sexual intercourse	197	89.5
Threatened you to have sexual intercourse by any means	13	5.9
Physically forced you to have sexual intercourse	37	16.8
Tied you with a rope or something else in order to force you to have sexual intercourse.	2	0.9
Hit you first, then forced you to have sexual intercourse	7	3.2
PHYA (n=92)		
Beat or pushed you but without trauma or persistent pain or limited movement in some parts of your body	86	93.5
Hit you with fists, kicked or cut you, with persistent pain or limited movement in some parts of your body	17	18.5
Beat you, leading to serious contusion, burn or fracture	0	0.0
Head or viscera trauma, permanent injury.	3	3.3
Injured you with tools or a weapon	5	2.3

2.4 Geographical differences in domestic violence

The surveys show a significant difference in prevalence of domestic violence depending on the area (P <0.002). Domestic violence, and other forms of violence, was most prevalent in Henan Province, followed by Shannxi Province. Prevalence was significantly higher in Henan than in Tianjing and Liaoning (P< 0.05) (see Table 28).

Table 28. Prevalence of domestic violence, by area

Area	Domestic violence (%)	PSYA (%)	SEXA (%)	PHYA (%)
Henan (299)	88 (29.4)	13 (4.3)	68 (22.7)	34 (11.4)
Shannxi (303)	74 (24.4)	10 (3.3)	59 (19.5)	26 (8.6)
Tianjing (300)	56 (18.7)	6 (2.0)	47 (15.7)	12 (4.0)
Liaoning (313)	56 (17.9)	8 (2.6)	46 (14.7)	20 (6.4)

2.5 Reasons for physical abuse

One-third of the women who had suffered physical violence reported no special reason as to why their partners had abused them. Other reasons given included lack of money, partners being perceived as unfaithful by their wives, partners being unhappy because of their jobs, or partners being drunk.

One-third of the perpetrators had promised to stop the abuse, but had not complied with their promises.

2.6 Women's actions after physical abuse

Most of the women said they had struck back when abused by their partners (23% every time, 33.7% occasionally).

Almost half (49.4%) had not told anyone about the abuse, while more than one-quarter said they had told friends or family members.

Nearly three-quarters (73.7%) of the women reported that they were suffering psychosomatic problems due to their partners' abuse, and one-quarter of them felt the effects to be severe.

3. Factors related to domestic violence

3.1 Sociodemographic characteristics of abused and non-abused women

The sociodemographic characteristics of the women (abused and non-abused groups) in the study, and of their intimate partners (perpetrator and non-perpetrator groups), are shown in Tables 29 and 30.

The sociodemographic characteristics of the abused and non-abused women were compared using χ^2 and T-test statistic analyses, but no significant differences were found between the two groups. A similar result was found in comparing perpetrator and non-perpetrator groups.

Table 29. Sociodemographic characteristics of abused and non-abused women

Sociodemographic characteristic	Abused (n=274) N (%)	Non-abused (n=941) N (%)	P
Age (years)			0.69
<20	14 (5.1)	39 (4.1)	
20-30	187 (68.2)	670 (71.2)	
31-40	67 (24.5)	207 (22.0)	
>40	6 (2.2)	25 (2.7)	
Educational level			0.86
Primary school	7 (2.6)	23 (2.4)	
Junior high school	58 (21.2)	178 (18.9)	
Senior high school	106 (38.7)	368 (39.1)	
University / above	103 (37.6)	371 (39.5)	
Occupation			0.58
White-collar worker	111 (40.5)	399 (42.4)	
Blue-collar worker	163 (59.5)	542 (57.6)	
Monthly income (Yuan)			0.62
<300	58 (21.2)	219 (23.3)	
301-800	113 (41.2)	396 (42.1)	
>800	103 (37.6)	326 (34.6)	
Marriage			0.75
First marriage	207 (75.5)	709 (75.3)	
Remarried	5 (1.8)	11 (1.2)	
Single	60 (21.9)	217 (23.1)	
Divorced	2 (0.7)	4 (0.4)	
Smoke			0.71
Yes	25 (9.1)	79 (8.4)	
No	249 (90.9)	862 (91.6)	
Drink			0.67
Yes	59 (21.5)	214 (22.7)	
No	215 (78.5)	727 (77.3)	
Drugs			0.77
Yes	4 (1.5)	12 (1.3)	
No	270 (98.5)	928 (98.7)	

Table 30. Sociodemographic characteristics of male perpetrators and non-perpetrators

Sociodemographic characteristics	Perpetrator(n=274) N (%)	Non-perpetrator(n=941) N (%)	P
Age (years)			0.12
<20	6 (2.2)	10 (1.1)	
20-30	159 (58.0)	595 (63.2)	
31-40	96 (35.0)	278 (29.5)	
>40	13 (4.7)	58 (6.2)	
Educational level			0.28
Primary school	8 (2.9)	14 (1.5)	
Junior high school	52 (19.0)	158 (16.8)	
Senior high school	93 (33.9)	355 (37.8)	
University / above	121 (44.2)	413 (43.9)	
Occupation			0.74
White-collar worker	120 (43.8)	423 (45.0)	
Blue-collar worker	154 (56.2)	518 (55.0)	
Monthly income (Yuan)			0.538
<300	15 (5.5)	69 (7.3)	
301-800	85 (31.0)	277 (29.4)	
>800	174 (63.5)	595 (63.2)	
Smoke			0.79
Yes	204 (74.4)	692 (73.5)	
No	70 (25.6)	249 (26.5)	
Drink			0.21
Yes	220 (80.3)	722 (76.7)	
No	54 (19.7)	219 (23.3)	
Drugs			1.000*
Yes	5 (1.8)	17 (1.8)	
No	269 (98.2)	923 (98.2)	

*: Fisher's Exact Test

3.2 History of pregnancy termination and other relevant factors

The average number of abortions among the abused women seeking pregnancy termination was 1.2, significantly higher than that of the non-abused women (0.86) ($p<0.001$). As shown in Table 31, the proportion of abused women who had undergone multiple assisted abortions was statistically significantly higher than for the non-abused women. No difference was found between the two groups regarding spontaneous abortions.

There was no difference between the abused and non-abused groups in the proportion using contraception.

Also, no differences were found between the two groups regarding abortion decision-making and willingness to have an abortion.

Table 31. History of abortions and related factors

Items	Abused (n=274) N (%)	Non-abused (n=941) N (%)	P
Number of abortions			0.000#
0	90 (32.8)	432 (45.9)	
1	107 (39.1)	334 (35.5)	
>1	77 (28.1)	175 (18.6)	
Number of spontaneous abortions			0.307
0	251 (91.6)	883 (93.8)	
1	16 (5.8)	45 (4.8)	
>1	7 (2.6)	13 (1.4)	
Reasons for current pregnancy			0.921
Failure of contraceptive use	115 (42.0)	396 (42.1)	
No contraceptive used	159 (58.0)	545 (57.9)	
Decision-making for abortion			0.666
Partner attending	257 (93.8)	895 (95.1)	
Partner not attending	9 (3.3)	27 (2.9)	
Partner unknown	8 (2.9)	19 (2.0)	
Willingness to have abortion			0.298
Willing	214 (78.1)	748 (79.5)	
Unwilling, compelled by partner	3 (1.1)	22 (2.3)	

\# P<0.05

The primary reasons given for choosing pregnancy termination were compared between the abused and non-abused groups (Table 32).

"Relationship with partner" was significantly more likely to be stated as the reason for abortion by women with a history of abuse than by non-abused women ($P<0.001$).

There were also significant differences between the two group in choosing "already have a child" and "taking harmful medicine" as reasons for termination.

Table 32. Reasons for pregnancy termination

Reasons	Abused (n=274) N (%)	Non-abused (n=941) N (%)	P
Already have a child	123 (44.9)	333 (35.4)	0.004#
Unmarried	43 (15.7)	146 (15.5)	0.948
Untimely	26 (9.5)	90 (9.6)	0.966
Taking harmful medicine	17 (6.2)	98 (10.4)	0.036#
Occupation / study	14 (5.1)	57 (6.1)	0.554
Financial	7 (2.6)	45 (4.8)	0.108
Relationship with partner	5 (1.8)	1 (0.1)	0.000*#
Not in a good mood	1 (0.4)	6 (0.6)	0.599*
Drinking too much	1 (0.4)	4 (0.4)	0.890*
In contact with harmful goods	1 (0.4)	3 (0.3)	0.907*
Family pressure	0	1 (0.1)	/

* Fisher's Exact Test; \# P<0.05

3 Comparison of life experience related to domestic violence

The abused women were more likely to have witnessed parental violence than the non-abused women. Also, 13.1% of the partners of women who had experienced violence had witnessed domestic violence in their own homes. However, only 5.3% of the partners of women who had never been abused had witnessed domestic violence in their homes. There is thus a statistically significant difference between the two groups. In addition, compared with non-abused women, more abused women knew of domestic violence against wives and girlfriends in their friendship networks and neighbourhoods (see Table 33).

Table 33. Experience of domestic violence among women seeking abortions

Experience	Abused (n =274) N (%)	Non-abused (n=941) N (%)	P
Witnessed parents' violence as a child			0.000
No	180 (65.7)	726 (77.2)	
Yes	77 (28.1)	160 (17.0)	
Know partner's father beats his wife			0.000
No	122 (44.5)	510 (54.2)	
Yes	36 (13.1)	50 (5.3)	
Know someone (wife/girlfriend) who is beaten			0.000
No	72 (26.3)	325 (34.5)	
Yes	173 (63.1)	465 (49.4)	

3.4 Relationship with partner

There were highly significant differences between the abused and non-abused groups regarding their relationships with their partners (see Table 34). The abused women had more limitations on their economic and personal freedom, and worse relationships with their partners.

The proportion of women who quarreled with their partners was also higher in the abused group than in the non-abused group. The abused women were significantly more likely to suffer their partners' neglect and indifferent treatment, and 23.4% of them were not allowed to control money freely, compared with 12.2% of the non-abused women (P<0.001).

Table 34. Relationship with partner, comparing abused and non-abused women seeking pregnancy termination

Relationship with partner	Abused (n =274) N (%)	Non-abused (n=941) N (%)	P Value
Are you afraid of your partner?			0.001
Never	217 (79.2)	821 (87.2)	
Sometimes	50 (18.2)	112 (11.9)	
Often	7 (2.6)	8 (0.9)	
How often do you quarrel with your partner?			0.000
Never	64 (22.6)	398 (42.2)	
Sometimes	188 (69.3)	518 (55.2)	
Often	22 (8.1)	25 (2.6)	
Does your partner ignore you and treat you indifferently?			0.000
Never	164 (59.9)	733 (77.9)	
Sometimes	103 (37.6)	206 (21.9)	
Often	7 (2.6)	2 (0.2)	
Does your partner damage your treasures or pets on purpose?			0.002
Never	236 (86.1)	874 (92.9)	
Sometimes	37 (13.5)	64 (6.8)	
Often	1 (0.4)	3 (0.3)	
If you talk to another man, does your partner get angry?			0.000
Never	126 (46.0)	565 (60.0)	
Sometimes	127 (46.4)	359 (38.2)	
Often	21 (7.7)	17 (1.8)	
If you need some money, is your partner always reluctant to give it to you?			0.000
Never	210 (76.6)	825 (87.8)	
Sometimes	60 (21.9)	95 (10.1)	
Often	4 (1.5)	21 (2.2)	

3.5 Effects of domestic violence on women's psychosomatic health

Tables 35 and 36 show the psychosomatic health of the two groups. Although the prevalence rates of upper reproductive tract infection and anaemia were higher in the abused group, the differences were not statistically significant. However, the results do show a statistically significant difference in the prevalence of lower reproductive tract infection between women who had suffered physical abuse and those who had not.

The Self-rating Depression Scale was used to screen the women for depression problems, with the results showing a higher prevalence in the abused group. As Table 36 shows, there were statistically significant differences in rates of medium and severe depression between the two groups.

Table 35. Prevalence of diseases among women seeking pregnancy termination

	Abused (n=274) N (%)	Non abused (n=941) N (%)	P
Upper RTI (Pelvic inflammatory disease)	18 (6.6)	47 (5.0)	0.980
Lower RTI (Cervicitis, vaginitis)	83 (30.3)	198 (21.0)	0.205
Anaemia	39 (14.2)	117 (12.4)	0.871

Table 36. Depression among women seeking pregnancy termination

Degree of depression	Abused (n=274) N (%)	Non abused (n=941) N (%)
Light	69 (25.2)	230 (24.4)
Medium	45 (16.4)	96 (10.2)#
Severe	12 (4.4)	18 (1.9)*

\# $P<0.01$; * <0.05

3.6 Seeking help after domestic violence

When the women were asked who they would turn to for help first if they encountered domestic violence, the first five answers in order of magnitude were: family members, friends, would not tell anyone, policemen and the village committee. There was a significantly higher proportion who chose "would not tell anyone" in the abused group than in the non-abused group (35.0% vs 14.6%, p<0.05).

To sum up the results, the respondents were generally younger and at lower educational and economic levels than their partners. The prevalence of domestic violence was not lower than in other relevant research findings, but there were significant differences in domestic violence prevalence rates depending on the survey area. Also, sexual violence was found to be the most common type of domestic violence. After using the χ^2, T-test statistic and Fisher exact test analysis, it was found that there are associative relationships between domestic violence and 11 variables: the number of abortions, depression, both the women and their partners witnessing their fathers beating their mothers in childhood, living in an environment with wife abuse, being afraid of partners, quarrelling with partners, suffering partners' indifference or estrangement, partners always intentionally damaging the women's favourite belongings, partner's becoming angry if the women had contact with other males, and the partners controlling the money.

CONCLUSIONS

1. Domestic violence among women seeking abortions

The survey revealed that 22.6% of the women seeking pregnancy termination had suffered domestic violence, which is similar to the findings of Evins and Chescheir's 1996 study (21.6%) and a little lower than the level found in Leung's study (27.3%) in Hong Kong in 1999[111,112]. However, their cultural background could have prohibited some abused women from disclosing their experience of abuse and seeking help in domestic violence screening or agreeing to participate in a survey. As stated above, traditional Chinese customs have taught women that family affairs should not be exposed to those outside the family. Therefore, the actual prevalence of domestic violence is likely to have been underestimated because some abused women did not participate in the research.

The survey also shows that the damage resulting from domestic violence was perceived by most abused women to be mild and not the cause of serious injury. Such a situation accords with the invisibility of domestic violence and the fact that it is easily ignored by others, including the authorities charged with dealing with it.

2. Sexual violence within the family

Sexual violence within the family includes marital rape. Western scientists in the 1970s identified marital rape as one of main forms of domestic violence of the twentieth century and suggested that, although seriously underreported, the number of marital rapes far exceeded non-marital rapes. In 2000, Guo recorded the results of a survey carried out in China among 4049 women, 113 of whom admitted to having been raped by their husbands[113]. His research found that sexual violence was the most common type of domestic violence, with a prevalence rate of 18% (220). Among the women who had been abused physically, 45.7% of them had also suffered sexual abuse. Previous studies show prevalence rates ranging from 4% to 33.5%, the differences possibly arising from the different measurement scales used.[114,115,116]

Since sexual activity between spouses has been always considered private, and husbands have traditionally had a legal right to have sex with their wives, it is difficult to measure marital rape. It is kept even more underground than general domestic violence, and has so far not been included in law in the majority of countries in the world. In countries where it has been criminalized, such the Philippines, authorities only rarely act on the law or intervene.

However, marital rape damages women's psychosomatic health and may cause sexual indifference or fear of sex[117]. The present survey revealed that unwanted pregnancy is related significantly to sexual abuse or marital rape, a finding similar to previous studies[118,119,120]. Research reports that victims of sexual violence within the family may have a higher prevalence of unwanted pregnancy because they often have difficulty in accessing and using proper and effective contraception. Therefore, it is necessary to conduct further research on policies and interventions for sexual violence within the family.

---

[111] *Op cit.* Ref 23.
[112] *Op cit.* Ref 75.
[113] Wu Changzhen. Summarization of domestic violence studies. In: China Law Society, Institution of Marriage and Family in China People University, England Cultural Committee, editors. Research on Domestic Violence Prevention. Beijing: Mass Press, 2000. P. 13-16.
[114] Wiebe ER, Janssen P. Universal screening for domestic violence in abortion. *Women's Health Issues*, 2001 Sept-Oct, 11(5):436-41.
[115] Kaye D. Domestic violence and induced abortion: report of three cases. *East Afr Med J.*, 2001 Oct, 78(10):555-6.
[116] *Op cit.* Ref 23.
[117] *Op cit.* Ref 2.
[118] Petersen R, Gazmararian J, et al. Partner violence: implications for health and community settings. *Women's Health Issues*, 2001, 11:116-25.
[119] Op cit. Ref 115.
[120] Domestic violence. ACOG issues technical bulletin on domestic violence. American College of Obstetricians and Gynecologists. *American Family Physician*, 1995 Dec, 52(8):2387-8, 2391.

3. Potential risk factors related to domestic violence

The survey found that the following factors were significantly associated with domestic violence against women.

3.1 Quarrelling with partners

Quarrelling itself may result in psychological and emotional harm to both women and men, especially when verbal threats are made and acted upon. The survey shows that quarrelling with partners is a major risk factor for physical and sexual abuse. In Chinese traditional culture, quarrels between spouses or intimate partners are considered private and should never become public. However, given the close association between quarrelling and domestic violence, social workers and other frontline health and welfare professionals should not neglect the significance of quarrelling between women seeking help and their partners. Those workers and professionals at the 'coalface' of health and welfare are in a good position to advocate for the issue of troubled, quarrelling marriage partners to be converted into a public issue, with implications for law, policy and service provision, including early intervention.

3.2 Suffering partners' indifference or estrangement.

Some researches have regarded indifference as a type of domestic violence. However, the current survey designates it as a risk factor. The survey results show that indifference or estrangement on the part of a partner is closely associated with all three types of domestic violence. Women who suffer their partners' indifference or estrangement are therefore certainly at risk.

3.3 Partners' unhappiness when women talk with other men.

The proportion of partners unhappy about their wives talking to other men was higher in the abused group than in the non-abused group, indicating that some partners are still influenced by traditional Chinese patriarchal culture. They regard their wives / girlfriends as their own private property, and do not allow them to have contact with other males for fear of them being regarded as "unfaithful". Essentially, women are treated as their partners' property and asked to obey men absolutely. This taboo against speaking to other men was one of the key factors leading to domestic violence among those surveyed.

3.4 Partners always unwilling to give money to women when they need it.

This is a kind of economic control of women, and has been included in some definitions of domestic violence and sometimes regarded as a type of domestic violence. Economic control shows, not only that men are unwilling to give their partners money, but also reflects the fact that the economic power of women is weaker than that of men and that women have to depend on men totally, even if they are wage-earners themselves.

3.5 Life experience of domestic violence

The risk of domestic violence is increased if men have come from families with domestic violence or if women are living in an environment with high levels of domestic violence. This is consistent with the theory that domestic violence is learnt from direct experience or observation. Males learn domestic violence from their childhood experiences of wife abuse and discover that domestic violence can have benefits (mothers obey husbands, wives obey husbands, or bad emotions are released) without any punishment. Therefore, they learn domestic violence as an adaptive response and gradually it becomes part of their customary behaviour.

3.6 Effects of domestic violence on women's physical and mental health

Many research studies have consistently found that domestic violence can damage women's mental health[121,122,123]. The results of the study indicate a significantly higher prevalence of depression in the abused group, including higher rates of medium or severe depression, proving that domestic violence does indeed harm women's social, mental and emotional health.

The prevalence of reproductive tract infections in the abused group was also significantly higher than in the non-abused group, but no difference was found between the sexually abused group and the non-sexually abused group, implying that the research hypothesis is not valid. It could be that the women's incorrect recollections contributed to lower reported prevalence of reproductive tract infections than was actually the case. The relationship between sexual violence and prevalence of RTIs should be studied further.

CHAPTER 6.
MEN'S ACCOUNTS OF DOMESTIC VIOLENCE

This chapter presents the results of focus groups discussions that were held with men to gain an understanding of their views on domestic violence.

RESULTS

1. Perceptions of a good husband

The men thought that a good husband should take responsibility for his family and should take care of the other members of the family. The ultimate authority of the husband was commonly recognized by the men in the focus groups.

2. Perceptions of a good wife

According to the men's perspective, a good wife should understand her husband. She should focus on her husband, children and family, and should show respect to the elderly. However, some of the men thought that men and women should have equal rights and that men should also have some responsibility for doing housework.

> *In my opinion, a good wife can take good care of family members, including my parents. That is all.*

> *I have a different opinion. Nowadays, women and men are equal. No matter if a man or a woman, all have the responsibility of taking care of the family.*

3. Attitudes towards gender roles

The majority of the men said they believed that "men should be responsible for external affairs and women should be responsible for domestic affairs". They said it was difficult to change that traditional belief. A man is the head of his family and should dominate his wife. The men also believed that they would lose face if women were responsible for external affairs. So in the traditional model, capable

---

[121] *Op cit.* Ref 1.
[122] *Op cit.* Ref 2.
[123] *Op cit.* Ref 3.

men marry weak women. If a woman was more capable than her husband, the old pattern would be disturbed and the position of the man, as head of the family, would be shaken, and the family would not be stable. The men found this unacceptable.

> *My position should be higher than my wife's. If she is a manager, I will be a general manager. I would let her down if my position could not become higher than hers.*

The majority of the men believed that small domestic affairs could be decided by the wife, but big ones must be decided by the husband. Some men thought that the wife could not decide anything by herself.

> *She does not have the capability to make a decision by herself, even if I let her do so. She usually doesn't have any idea until I make the decision.*

> *I would be angry if my wife bought a big television without my permission.*

However, there were also some educated men in the focus group who thought this an archaic traditional gender role. They argued that, nowadays, men and women have equal rights. Therefore, both women and men should be responsible for external and domestic affairs, especially when many people are unemployed. They suggested that it did not matter whether a man or a woman, taking responsibility for external affairs should depend on the couple's personal capacities.

I would prefer to do housework at home if my wife earned more money than me.

4. Perceptions of gender-related violence

4.1 Attitudes towards physical abuse

The men were asked to give their opinions on the different types of physical abuse listed in Table 37. About half of them thought that hitting or punching and throwing objects at their wives did not constitute abuse. About 40% thought that shutting their wives out of their homes was not abuse, even if it involved punching. The majority of the men thought that the other types of behaviour on the list did constitute physical abuse (see Table 37).

Table 37. Attitudes towards physical abuse

Type of behaviour	Believe to be abuse	Percentage (%)
1. Hitting or punching her	17	45
2. Throwing objects at her	21	55
3. Shutting her out of the home	23	62
4. Punching her out of the home	24	63
5. Refusing to help her when she is ill	32	84
6. Discarding her in a dangerous /wild area	32	86
7. Beating or punishing her	33	87
8. Slapping or biting her	34	89
9. Kicking or choking her	36	95
10. Threatening to harm her with a weapon	37	97

4.2 Attitudes towards emotional abuse

The men's opinions about emotional abuse were collected by questionnaire. About half of them thought that being angry with their wives for talking to other men and controlling their wives' spending money were not abuse. About 40% thought that treating their wives with indifference, blaming them for being unfaithful or ignoring their emotions were not abuse (see Table 38).

Table 38. Attitude towards emotional abuse

Type of behaviour	Believe to be abuse	Percentage (%)
Being angry if she talks to another man	16	42
Controlling her spending money	20	54
Ignoring her or treating her with indifference	22	58
Blaming her for being unfaithful	22	58
Ignoring her emotions	23	60
Threatening to separate her baby from her	27	71
Damaging her treasures or pets on purpose	28	74
Forbidding her to contact her family members and friends	29	76
Often insulting her	32	84
Often sneering and humiliating her	33	87
Threatening to hit her	34	92

5. Reasons for battering

A minority of the men in the focus group said that they believed that a man should not batter his wife under any circumstances, no matter whether the wife makes a mistake or not. However, the majority thought that a man has a right to batter his wife under the following circumstances: (1) if she curses the husband in public or on other occasions that could cause loss of the husband's dignity; (2) for not respecting her parents-in-law; or (3) if the wife is having an extramarital affair.

They also believed that battering is a sign of a man's intimacy with his wife and cursing shows the wife that her husband loves her. Some men seemed to construct their violence as a rational response to extreme provocation, resulting in loss of control. They said that, in most circumstances, a wife is responsible for her husband's violent behavior because women are "always garrulous", which is harmful to men's mental health. Thus wife battering is seen as an inevitable outcome of nagging. In fact, the men said that they were on the receiving end of more emotional abuse than women.

> *I couldn't tolerate my wife's babbling. Sometimes I ran away. But occasionally, it was too boring, I beat her.*

> *I think that the women must have had some faults. They wouldn't be beaten without an apparent reason.*

Some men believed that wife battering is rare in the city, but common in rural areas. They also thought that wife battering only occurred in populations with low levels of education or in couples with big gaps in level of education. Some men thought wives should obey their husbands under any circumstance, otherwise, they should be punished by force.

> *My wife never obeyed my suggestions. What should I do? She always talked more until I beat her. I thought wife battering was very common among my friends.*

6. Handling the matter after wife battering

The majority of the men believed that a couple's fighting was a private matter and should be handled by the couple. No one else should interfere. If an outsider interfered, the men thought it would mean a loss of face for them as men, which might lead to further battering. The men perceived battering and quarrelling between couples as the norm.

> *When the screams were heard, people went out. When we found out that it was only a couple beating each other, all the people went. Therefore, the couple could freely beat each other.*

> *I saw a fight between the couple who are my neighbours. I wanted to intervene because they are my friends. However, they said it was a private matter. No one could interfere with it.*

> *Wife battering should not be interfered with unless someone's life is in danger. We rarely come to settle husband-and-wife beating cases. This is family business.*

CONCLUSIONS

1. Men believe that only the severe end of the scale is domestic violence

The results show that the majority of men only think of hitting, biting, kicking, slapping or threatening with weapons as domestic violence. Some men do not recognize other kinds of behaviour, especially behaviour that causes emotional harm, as domestic violence. Such findings indicate that educational programmes on domestic violence should be delivered through the mass media and should be directed at men as well as women.

2. The 'big man' attitude is still common among men, although attitudes are changing.

Although men and women are equal under Chinese law, the traditional belief of being a 'big man' is still common in the majority of men. Some men think their position at home must be higher than women's. Otherwise, they would lose face. The men believe that a wife must obey her husband. If not, the husband has the right to maintain his position at home by force. However, nowadays, some men's attitudes are changing, which gives some hope to the possibility of preventing domestic violence against women. The challenge is to convert attitudes to behaviour.

3. Men see their violence as a rational response to extreme provocation, a loss of control, and see their wives as being responsible for their behaviour.

Domestic violence against women, which seems to be the outbreak of unsatisfied emotion, highlights the inequality between couples and the lower status of women at home. It also indicates that some men do not have the capacity to cope appropriately with conflicts.

4. Men regard domestic violence as a private issue.

The majority of the men in the focus groups said that they regarded domestic violence as a private matter and believed that no one else should interfere. General public opinion in China also regards domestic violence as a private issue and something which is acceptable in the husband and wife relationship. That is why such violence can persist.

CHAPTER 7.
MATERNAL AND CHILD HEALTH WORKERS' KNOWLEDGE, ATTITUDES AND PRACTICES REGARDING DOMESTIC VIOLENCE

Domestic violence against women has become a major public health problem. Health practitioners do not screen for it at clinics and there is a serious lack of appropriate intervention measures, which is the biggest obstacle to supporting abused women. What is the use of identifying cases of domestic violence when there are no services to which to direct either the male perpetrators or the female survivors? However, getting health practitioners to recognize domestic violence as a public health issue is the first step in encouraging them to become advocates for improved governmental and nongovernmental services for both perpetrators and survivors. In this chapter, an attempt is made to understand health practitioners' knowledge, attitudes and practices with regard to domestic violence.

RESULTS

1. Sociodemographic characteristics of respondents

The sample consisted of 139 health practitioners working in the area of maternal and child health. The age of the respondents ranged from 21 to 55 years, with a mean of 40 years. In the sample, 8 participants (5.8%) were male and 131 (94.2%) were female, and the majority (67.2%) had graduated from college or above. They were from provincial hospitals (10.8%), city hospitals (22.3%), and country hospitals (66.9%), nearly three-quarters of them (76.4%) maternal and child health hospitals. Among the respondents, 68.4% were maternal and child health workers and 16.2% were child health care workers, while 15.4% were other health personnel. Their years of work experience ranged from 1 to 38, with a mean of 17 years.

2. Knowledge and attitudes towards domestic violence

Nearly one-third (31.4%) of the health practitioners in the sample did not consider domestic violence a medical issue, and more than four-fifths said that they were more qualified in dealing with physical health. Most of them (68.6%) thought that there were much more important things to ask patients about than domestic violence. More than one-third (35.8%) said that they had no time to make enquiries or assess the situation regarding domestic violence, and more than half (61.4%) felt incompetent to deal with domestic violence victims. More than one-quarter (28%) of the respondents believed that if they asked patients questions related to domestic violence, the patients would become angry with them. About one-tenth of them did not care about patients' domestic violence (see Table 39).

Table 39. Knowledge and attitudes towards domestic violence

	Agree	Not sure	Disagree
1. Domestic violence does not occur in the middle or upper classes.	60.4	29.5	10.1
2. Some women are responsible for domestic violence.	12.4	19.0	68.6
3. I do not care about patients' domestic violence.	10.8	17.4	71.8
4. Domestic violence is not a medical issue.	31.4	21.9	46.7
5. I am qualified to deal with physical health only.	84.1	10.1	5.8
6. Patients would be angry with me if I asked them about domestic violence.	28.0	42.5	29.5
7. There are much more important things to ask patients about than domestic violence.	68.6	16.8	14.6
8. I have no time to make enquiries and assessments about domestic violence.	35.8	21.9	42.3
9. I am incompetent to deal with domestic violence.	61.4	12.4	26.12

3. Practices

Almost all (92.1%) the respondents said they did not enquire routinely about domestic violence, although four-fifths (80%) of them said they saw victims in their clinical practices. Nearly three-quarters (72.2%) said they did not provide any help for victims. Even although patients told them about long-term discomfort, sexual problems and chronic pelvic infections, 63.1% of the respondents said they did not enquire about domestic violence. Nine-tenths (90%) had never been trained on domestic violence, and most (97%) thought such training necessary.

CONCLUSIONS

Health practitioners do not enquire routinely about abuse or document abuse as the cause of their patients' symptoms, despite the fact that they see victims of domestic violence in their clinical practices. They feel incompetent to deal with domestic violence and believe they need training on the topic. Therefore, it is necessary to develop a continuing education programme to train health practitioners on domestic violence.

Chapter 8.
RECOMMENDATIONS

1. In-depth training and awareness-raising for all health professionals

Training health care professionals about the problems of domestic violence is a critical and necessary first step in early identification and intervention efforts. Advocates should turn attention toward reforming the response of health care providers to victims of abuse. However, the study found that doctors rarely ask a female patient whether she is being abused, even when there are obvious signs of violence.

It is clear that many health professionals do not consider it appropriate to ask about domestic violence in a clinical setting. The failure of health professionals to identify domestic violence and offer appropriate interventions has been attributed to a number of factors including lack of knowledge and adequate training, lack of time, fear of offending the women, fear of opening up issues which could get out of control, a belief that domestic violence is not the province of health professionals, and a feeling of being powerless to 'fix' the situation.

Therefore, health care interventions should focus on sensitizing providers, encouraging routine screening for abuse, and institutionalizing protocols for the proper management of abuse.

2. Identification and disclosure of domestic violence in health settings

Most women are likely to interact with the health system at some point in their lives: when they seek contraception or give birth. Pregnancy is one of the only times that healthy women have frequent, scheduled contact with health service providers. This makes the health care setting an important venue to identify women experiencing abuse and provide them with needed support and referral. Pregnancy is a time when society offers support to a woman so that she may bring a healthy baby into the world. The possible health consequences for both the mother and her unborn child may motivate women to seek help or take steps to leave an abusive relationship. In addition, the trusting relationship that develops between the patient and the doctor can be a powerful vehicle for guiding behavioural change. Therefore, the prenatal clinic is a good place to screen for domestic violence and start interventions, as well as seek out appropriate referral.

Screening refers to routine enquiry about domestic violence of all women using maternity services. Studies in maternity settings have shown that the use of repeated screening and a structured screening questionnaire increases the rate of detection of domestic violence significantly[124,125,126].

This study also suggests that abuse should be considered a factor contributing to poor obstetric outcomes.

3. Multisectoral cooperation

An interdisciplinary, multi-agency approach is the most effective way of addressing domestic violence. Different sectors, such as the police, health services, the judiciary and social support services (governmental and nongovernmental) must work together in order to meet the range of needs that women in violent relationships experience. Otherwise, the health sector's action will be useless.

---

[124] *Op cit.* Ref 69.
[125] Norton LB *et al*. Battering in pregnancy: An assessment of two screening methods. *Obstetrics and Gynecology*, 1995, 85:321-325.
[126] *Op cit.* Ref 16.

4. Development of an education and counselling system for prevention of domestic violence

It is necessary to develop an education and counselling system for prevention of domestic violence using the following means:

(a) **Intensify publicity.**

(b) **Establish favorable circumstances for the protection of women's rights and elimination of domestic violence in all sectors of society.** It is necessary to educate all members of society to change society's perceptions and attitudes. Ending domestic violence against women means changing substantially the perceptions, attitudes and beliefs that are traditionally held in communities and society as a whole. Only when society's perception of domestic violence changes, can large-scale, society-wide responses to violence take place. All members of society (men, women and children) must be educated on gender roles, to fight violence against women and to respect each citizen's social, economic, human and bodily rights. It should be explained that violent behaviour, cruelty and inhumanity are illegal acts at the national level, and contravene international conventions at the global level.

(c) **Educate men.** Men should be educated about gender equality and sharing responsibility in marriage, family matters and decision-making with their wives. In addition, information, education and communication programmes should provide information about the adverse reproductive health consequences of domestic violence, especially domestic violence during pregnancy.

(d) **Educate and empower women.** It is necessary to educate women about gender roles and reactions to any type of domestic violence. Pre-marriage check-ups in China provide a good chance to educate the couple before marriage. Therefore, education on domestic violence and gender roles should be integrated into pre-marriage health education programmes.

(e) **Equip family, friends and communities to respond constructively to domestic violence.** Since many women will never access 'official' services or systems, it is very important to expand informal sources of support through neighbourhood and friendship networks, communities and workplaces. Most abused women reach out in the first instance to family members or friends, not formal institutions. How those individuals respond is highly predictive of whether a woman continues toward empowerment and action, or whether she retreats once again into isolation and self-blame. Therefore, it is necessary to have a programme aimed at combating harmful social norms that keep women trapped in abusive relationships, and to model more constructive responses to abuse on the part of family and friends.

(f) **Set up counselling centres or hotlines in rural areas to help battered women.** Although counselling centres and hotlines do exist in some big cities, it is difficult for rural people to access them. It is necessary to set up counselling centres and hotlines in rural areas to help battered women.

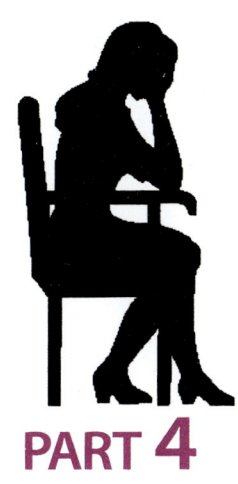

PART 4

MEDICO-LEGAL AND HEALTH SERVICES FOR VICTIMS OF SEXUAL VIOLENCE: A SITUATIONAL ANALYSIS IN THE PHILIPPINES

Table of Contents

Chapter 1. Introducion 115

Chapter 2. Background 115

Chapter 3. Study objectives 117

Chapter 4. Study methods 118

           Sampling strategy 119

           Limitations of the study 120

           Data analysis 120

Chapter 5. Study results 120

           Macro level 121

           Micro level 136

Chapter 6. Discussion 142

Chapter 7. Conclusions 143

Chapter 1. INTRODUCTION

Sexual violence constitutes a significant health and security concern that affects men and women throughout their lives. Studies conducted in various countries have found that up to 36% of girls and 29% of boys have suffered from sexual abuse. The magnitude of sexual coercion in adolescence is often similarly high: up to 46% of female and 20% of male adolescents have experienced coerced sex, depending on the country of study. Rape and domestic violence account for an estimated 5%-16% of the healthy years of life lost to women of reproductive age. Population-based studies report that between 12% and 25% of women have experienced attempted or completed forced sex by an intimate partner or ex-partner at some time in their lives.

Sexual violence has a significant impact on the physical and mental health of the victims. Its health consequences, among others, include unwanted pregnancy, genitourinary disorders, sexually transmitted infections, HIV/AIDS, mental health sequellae, self-inflicted injuries, and adoption of high-risk modes of behaviour, such as having multiple sexual partners and drug abuse.

The health care sector plays an important role in the recognition, documentation and response to individual cases of sexual assault. Persons who suffer from sexual violence often seek medical assistance, even without disclosure of the sexual assault, and are often taken to a health facility for examination after reporting an assault to the police. Health care workers can provide comprehensive, gender-sensitive health services to victims of sexual violence to help them to manage the physical and mental consequences of the assault. Such services include pregnancy testing, STI testing and prophylaxis, treatment of injuries, and psychosocial counselling. Related health assistance that may be provided to victims includes referrals to social welfare and legal aid, as well as collection and documentation of forensic evidence for the purposes of prosecution.

A panel of experts at the Consultation on Health Sector Response to Sexual Violence, organized by WHO in Geneva in June 2001, developed a series of health service objectives for the care of persons who have experienced sexual violence. These include:

- to improve health status;
- to ensure adequate documentation of evidence;
- to ensure satisfaction of client expectations; and
- to ensure involvement of the community.

Although it is recognized that there may be variation between countries in the formulation of service objectives, the WHO initiative on the health sector response to sexual violence has adopted these objectives as its guiding framework.

Chapter 2. BACKGROUND

This research was part of a proposal on research priorities developed by the Sexual Violence Research Initiative. It was taken up by WHO because it fitted within the organization's priorities for the development of normative guidance in the area of sexual violence. The proposal was for a study which would describe the structure and processes of sexual assault services in developing country settings, with the study results serving as the basis for the development of standards for good quality medico-legal and health services for persons who have experienced sexual violence.

In the Philippines, the magnitude of the sexual violence problem is a serious cause of concern. In 2001, the Philippine National Police recorded 7594 cases of sexual violence, 65% (4597) of which were committed against children and 35% (2637) against women.

In 1999, the University Center for Women's Studies (UCWS) and the Consuelo Zobel Alger Foundation completed a survey of 111 organizations in the Philippines that carry out various programmes for women and girls in difficult situations. The study showed that most of those programmes were concerned with the delivery of welfare services, education and health. There was a lack of legal assistance and a dearth of gender-sensitive and professionally-trained service providers. In 2002, UCWS again undertook a study, in cooperation with the Department of Health's Women's Health and Safe Motherhood Program, on selected cases of good practice in intervention programmes to prevent and eliminate violence against women and children. However, as far as the health care delivery system's response to the problem is concerned, there has been no systematic nationwide study to assess the practice and availability of medico-legal services for victims of sexual violence. This study is the first attempt to provide a situational analysis of medico-legal and health services available to persons who have experienced sexual violence.

In order to put such medico-legal and health services in the context of the current general health delivery system, a brief description of the health sector is needed. The Philippine health delivery system has been decentralized since health services were devolved to local governments in 1993, as mandated by the Local Government Code of 1991. Since that devolution, provincial and district hospitals have been operated and maintained by provincial or city governments, while rural health units, also known as municipal health offices, and *barangay* (village) health stations have been under the management of the municipal office. The latter two health facilities offer primary care, while secondary health care is offered at the level of the district or provincial hospitals. Because the local government units have autonomy in managing health service delivery in their areas of jurisdiction, there is no uniformity of health care across the country. However, in 1999, the Department of Health launched the '*Sentrong Sigla*' ('Centres of Vitality') movement, which fosters collaboration with the local government units in providing quality health services within a devolved health system. Under this programme, compliance with national standards set by Department of Health in eight areas earns the health unit the status of 'Centre of Vitality'.

There are different sets of standards for rural health units and *barangay* health centres, both of which are primary care facilities, and for the provincial/ city or district health hospitals. The eight areas of quality assessment are:

- infrastructure and amenities (clean water and functioning toilets);
- basic health services;
- attitudes and behaviour of health workers;
- human resources;
- equipment and laboratory capability;
- sufficient drugs, medicines and supplies;
- a health information system; and
- community intervention.

Basic health services include an expanded programme on immunization, disease surveillance, control of acute respiratory infection and diarrhoeal diseases, micronutrient supplementation/ nutrition, family planning, tuberculosis control, STI/ AIDS control and prevention, environmental sanitation, cervical cancer screening, and maternal care. Expected attitudes and behaviour of health workers include being women-friendly, as manifested by maintaining a women's desk at the hospital outpatient department and emergency room, among others. As of 2003, the Department of Health had awarded '*Sentrong Sigla*' status to 331 *barangay* health stations, 1394 rural health units and 97 district and provincial hospitals.

CHAPTER 3.
STUDY OBJECTIVES

The general study goal was to obtain data on the medico-legal and health services provided to victims of sexual violence through:

(1) documentation of the structure and resources of the health sector response to sexual violence; and

(2) documentation of the process of service delivery.

The specific study objectives were:

At the macro level:

(1) to identify any dedicated health services for persons who have experienced sexual violence, and to describe those services;

(2) to determine the nature of facilities providing sexual assault services, and to measure the number of facilities where services are provided and the number of services per 100 000 population;

(3) to determine which health workers provide forensic examination services and measure the number of trained forensic examiners per 100 000 population;

(4) to determine the duration, nature and content of basic training curricula for forensic examiners;

(5) to describe the geographical distribution of medico-legal services and determine the proportion of the population who do not live within 5km, 10km and 20km of a service;

(6) to identify policies on sexual assault and determine their availability at the facility level;

(7) to understand the organizational, financial and accountability structure of medico-legal services at national, provincial and district/regional levels and to describe the structure and nature of supervision and any accreditation system for medico-legal service providers;

(8) to determine the cost (and affordability) of accessing health services and medico-legal examination after sexual assault;

(9) to describe the extent to which the different needs of women, men and children who are victims of sexual violence are addressed in training, sexual assault policies and service provision;

(10) to describe the processes followed to maintain the chain of evidence and to package and transport evidence to laboratories; and

(11) to describe the number of laboratories available to carry out analysis of forensic evidence and the range of relevant services available in those laboratories.

At the micro (facility) level:

(1) to describe the physical infrastructure and equipment available at the facility level:

   (a) to describe the waiting area for examination, the post-examination waiting area and the facilities available for the examination, with particular emphasis on privacy and the procedures followed to prevent contact with the perpetrator; and

   (b) to describe the nature of the equipment and supplies (including medication) available at the facility level to provide medico-legal services to persons who have experienced sexual violence and to assess the adequacy of the equipment for the level of care provided;

(2) to assess the organizational structure of a representative sample of facilities and determine their links to external structures:

(a) to describe possible impediments to access to the facilities, including opening hours, after-hours arrangements, waiting times, disabled access, transport arrangements to and from the police, access to services in appropriate languages, acceptability of services, the extent to which health facilities are accessed prior to approaching the police, and whether victims are allowed access to care without going first to the police;

(b) to describe the mechanisms to guarantee the safety of service providers and clients and the frequency of problems of safety related to sexual assault care and the process of managing incidents;

(c) to assess the availability of information materials for patients on sexual assault, the examination, choices and sources of further support at the facility level; and

(d) to determine the existence and nature of accountability mechanisms for service users, sexual assault NGOs and the local community that are in place at the facility level;

(3) to describe the process of service provision in a representative sample of facilities and to assess the interpersonal dimension of service provision:

(a) to describe the attitudes of the staff providing sexual assault care towards sexual assault victims;

(b) to determine the nature of the interpersonal dimension of care, including the extent of information and choice provided to clients, the extent to which their rights are respected, and the availability of chaperones during service provision;

(c) to determine the number of sexual assault medico-legal examinations performed by staff providing this service per year;

(d) to describe problems encountered in collection of medico-legal evidence, including those related to rape kits (where available);

(e) to describe the proportion of examiners who have given evidence in court on sexual assault cases in the past year and the problems encountered;

(f) to describe indicators of the competence of staff providing sexual assault care, including pregnancy prevention and STI treatment, injury management, follow-up arrangements, psychological support, adequacy of documentation of forensic evidence;

(g) to assess the extent to which referrals to the police and sources of psychological support form part of the regular service provision process, and the nature of intersectoral relationships;

(h) to determine the satisfaction of clients with the services delivered and the main problems identified by clients with health services related to sexual assault; and

(i) to determine the use and familiarity of service providers with national, provincial and/or district policy on sexual violence, and whether they have been trained in its use.

CHAPTER 4.
STUDY METHODS

The study was carried out at two levels, the government level (national and provincial) and the facility level, using multiple research methods. The study methods were developed at an international meeting of experts sponsored by WHO, and were also based on the experience of the South African Gender-based Violence and Health Initiative, and the National Institute of Legal Medicine and Forensic Sciences in Bogotá, Colombia.

For the macro-level study, data were collected from the Department of Health and the National Bureau of Investigation through administration of a standard questionnaire, followed by face-to-face interviews.

The micro-level study was conducted at a representative sample of facilities in three sites: Manila, as the capital city, and Sorsogon and Oriental Mindoro, as the provinces chosen to represent under-resourced provinces in the country as a whole.

At the facility level, three data collection instruments were used: (1) a facility checklist of the availability and quality of the examination room, equipment and supplies; (2) a questionnaire addressed to service managers; and (3) a questionnaire administered to the service providers in the same facility. Interviews with client proxies represented by staff from other service organizations involved with sexual assault management, such as the police, the social welfare sector and NGOs, were also carried out to generate perspectives from service users of the health and medico-legal facilities.

SAMPLING STRATEGY

1. Overall sampling of study sites

Three sites were selected for the research exercise: Manila, as the capital city, and Sorsogon and Oriental Mindoro, as representative under-resourced provinces.

Based on the 2000 Family Income and Expenditures Survey, Sorsogon and Oriental Mindoro are among the 44 poorest provinces in the country. Both provinces are located in the Luzon islands, where more than half (56.0%) of the Philippine population resides. The remainder of the country's populace is almost equally distributed between the Mindanao (23.7%) and Visayas islands (20.3%).

The inaccessibility of the region and security concerns prevented the researchers from selecting study sites in the Visayan and Mindanao islands. On the other hand, the central Luzon provinces are regarded as industrialized or currently industrializing, while those in the upper north are generally mountainous and inaccessible.

Data on selected demographic indices among the three study sites and that of the country as a whole are relatively comparable (see Table 1).

Table 1. Comparison of demographic data: Philippines, Manila, Sorsogon and Oriental Mindoro, May 2000

Criteria	Philippines	Manila	Sorsogon	Oriental Mindoro
Population size	76 504 077	1 581 082	650 535	681 818
Population growth rate	2.36%	-0.97%	2.04%	2.46%
Average household size	5.0 persons	4.71 persons	5.19 persons	5.07 persons
Sex ratio	101.43	95.05	106.07	103.34
Dependency Ratio	69.04	50.81	86.08	81.64

The city of Manila accounts for 2.07% of the country's total population, while the two chosen provinces contribute relatively similar population proportions. Sorsogon shares 0.85% of the 76.5 million Philippine population and Oriental Mindoro, 0.89%.

As for average annual growth, the rate for Oriental Mindoro is slightly higher than the national value of 2.36%. The population growth rate for Sorsogon is much lower, and that of the capital city slowed down to –0.97% for the period 1995-2000.

In the two provinces, data on sex ratios suggest that there are more males for every 100 females, fairly similar to the national ratio of 101.43. On the other hand, females outnumber males in the city of Manila.

The dependency ratios for Sorsogon and Oriental Mindoro are much higher than those of the capital city and the whole country, and thus reflect the provinces' economic situation. This means that every 100 members of the economically productive age group (15-64 years) have to support more than 80 dependents (0-14 and 65+ years).

2. Macro level

Representatives who hold key positions in the Department of Health, the National Bureau of Investigation and the Philippine National Police were selected through convenience sampling and were interviewed using the standard questionnaires for the national and provincial levels.

3. Micro level

In order to obtain a sample of facilities in the three selected study sites, Manila, Sorsogon and Oriental Mindoro, the cluster sampling technique was employed. The health and/or medico-legal facility itself is regarded as the sampling unit or the unit of analysis. Such facilities include hospitals, primary health care clinics and specialty clinics that provide services concerned with sexual assault management.

A sampling frame, which included a list of such facilities, was created for each study site. From this, the sample to be included in the study was selected randomly in consultation with the guidelines provided in the research protocol.

In each site, three hospitals (one tertiary/regional hospital and two secondary/district hospitals) and one medico-legal facility (if applicable) were chosen at random from the list. Within the vicinity of these facilities, client proxies from other service organizations, such as a police officer, a social worker and an NGO representative, were also selected.

LIMITATIONS OF THE STUDY

Due to limited resources, the study was restricted to sampling only three provinces considered to be representative

DATA ANALYSIS

A database was constructed with Epi-Info 6 to compile the questionnaire results obtained from the closed-ended questions. A set of data analysis tables was provided to guide country investigators in the implementation of cross-tabulation of selected variables, and to ensure that common analysis was carried out throughout the country. Descriptive analysis was carried out for the results at the micro and macro levels. The open-ended questions were extracted and analysed through content analysis.

Data on the location and quantity of services was provided to a local centre specializing in the use of geographical information systems, which calculated the percentage of the population living within a radius of the facilities and mapped the availability of services.

Chapter 5.
STUDY RESULTS

A total of 81 respondents were interviewed for the study, 5 at the national/provincial and 76 at the facility level. Table 2 shows the breakdown of respondents.

Table 2. Respondent types by study site

Study site	Respondents						TOTAL
	National/Provincial representatives	Facility managers	Forensic examiners	Medical doctors	Registered nurses	Client proxies	
Manila	2	8	2	5	7	8	27
Oriental Mindoro	1	2	0	5	6	10	24
Sorsogon	2	3	0	6	6	13	30
TOTAL	5	8	2	16	19	31	81

This chapter presents and discusses the results of the macro-level and micro-level studies in separate sections. The former reflects the overview of services available and existing policies affecting the delivery of those services, while the latter reflects the actual implementation of the health and medico-legal services at the community level in three different regions of the country.

MACRO LEVEL

The leading national institutions that provide health and medico-legal (forensic) services to persons who have experienced sexual violence are the government-run hospitals under the Department of Health, the medico-legal facilities of the National Bureau of Investigation (NBI) and the Philippine National Police (PNP). The Department of Social Welfare and Development also runs community-based and institution-based programmes that offer crisis management and temporary shelter for the immediate protection of women in crisis. However, the Department of Social Welfare and Development coordinates with the Department of Health in providing health and medico-legal services to persons who have experienced sexual violence.

The services of the three leading institutions are described in detail below:

1. Department of Health

The Department of Health is part of the executive branch of the Government and is the lead agency for the health sector. Its mandate is to provide policy direction and plans for health programmes and services. With devolution to local governments, most direct services are now under the responsibility of the local government units, although the Department of Health maintains specialty centres, regional hospitals and medical centres. The responsibilities of the Department of Health include:

- health research and development;
- health surveillance and the health information system;
- resource generation for priority health services;
- technical assistance and logistical support to local health services;
- human resource capacity-building in health;
- health promotion and advocacy;
- direct service delivery for specialized health care;
- health care financing;
- health emergency preparedness and response;
- monitoring, assessment and evaluation of the health situation;
- quality assurance for health care; and
- networking for multisectoral actions on health.

The concept of a hospital-based crisis centre germinated in 1993 when the National Commission on the Role of Filipino Women convened a technical working group on violence against women, composed of nongovernmental organizations, such as the Women's Crisis Center, *PILIPINA, KALAKASAN, KANLUNGAN*, and the University of the Philippines Center for Integrative and Development Studies. The technical working group analysed the situation and eventually recommended multidisciplinary, multilevel responses to violence against women that included meeting the medical, legal, shelter and other psychosocial needs of victims. They also suggested collaboration between the women's NGOs that provide feminist crisis intervention services and the government agencies that can provide resources for the delivery of services. Thus was born Project HAVEN – Hospital Assisted Crisis Intervention for Women Survivors of a Violent Environment.

Project HAVEN became operational in 1995 under the leadership of the Women's Crisis Center, a women's NGO that pioneered crisis intervention for women survivors of abuse, in collaboration with the Department of Health. It was piloted at the East Avenue Medical Center, a government hospital in the National Capital Region. The project was later renamed Women and Children's Crisis Care and Protection Unit when it was institutionalized.

A year after the start of Project HAVEN's operations, the Department of Health piloted purely government-based Women's Desks in five government hospitals. In 1997, the then President of the Philippines, President Fidel V. Ramos, issued a memorandum entitled *A Call to Action against Domestic Violence*. That directive led to the issuance of an administrative order (AO No. 1-Bs) by the Department of Health mandating all hospitals retained by the Department to establish Women and Children Protection Units (WCPU).

To date, there are reported to be 44 WCPUs in the regional and specialty hospitals retained by the Department of Health all over the country. Seed funding was provided for the establishment of such facilities, but the funding for their continuous operation is shouldered by the respective hospitals. The WCPUs' goal is to provide holistic, gender-sensitive care to women and children who are victims of violence. The specific objectives are:

- to ensure that women and children who consult the Department of Health hospitals due to violence are **treated** with the utmost **care, concern and understanding (attitude);**

- to create and sustain an environment within the hospital setting that is **sensitive and friendly** to women and children (**attitude**);

- to develop a systematic, gender-sensitive **documentation and monitoring system**; and

- to **coordinate** with other governmental and nongovernmental institutions and organizations to achieve a more organized approach to address other, non-medical needs of victims of violence

Ideally, the WCPUs should have five main components in recognition of their multidisciplinary and collaborative approach to violence against women and children:

(1) **Medical, surgical, psychological and other health services** that feature 24-hour service, a holding and processing area for victims of violence, a standard clinical protocol for their examination and management, and a gender-sensitive recording system.

(2) **A networking mechanism** with other government organizations and NGOs to ensure an holistic and integrated approach to violence against women and children.

(3) **A training** programme that addresses human resource development, which the Department of Health undertakes with the University of the Philippines – Philippine General Hospital (UP-PGH) Child Protection Unit (CPU) and Women's Desk. (PGH, although a state hospital and considered the premier tertiary hospital in the country, is part of the University of the Philippines system. It is not directly under the Department of Health, and is therefore not counted amongst the 44 WCPUs of hospitals retained by the Department of Health.).

(4) **Research and documentation** of experiences to serve as input for further studies, policy and programme improvement.

(5) **Information and advocacy** campaigns by developing communication materials aimed at raising awareness about and preventing violence against women and children.

The WCPUs are supposed to be headed by the Chief of Clinics and staffed by an obstetrician-gynaecologist, a paediatrician, a nurse, a social worker and a psychiatrist, psychologist or counsellor. The gynaecologists, paediatricians and nurses are the ones usually sent by their respective hospitals to receive forensic training from the Government.

Most WCPUs may be classified as special examination suites, while three of the 44 centres are considered one-stop shops or national resource centres – one per major island group. These are the WCPUs in Baguio General Hospital (Northern Luzon), Vicente Sotto Memorial Medical Center (Central Visayas) and Davao Medical Center (Southern Mindanao).

The Department of Health has established the Women's Health and Development Program to provide technical assistance and policy direction to the WCPUs in the various hospitals it retains. The programme was established in 1998 with the aim of examining, not only biological, but also sociocultural factors, with a view to understanding the health needs of women. Its task is to ensure that all Department of Health programmes and services have a gender perspective.

The policies are disseminated to provincial authorities through the regional health offices of the Department. The Department of Health also provides technical assistance and training to local government units in their health programmes. Since health services are devolved from the provincial level down, Department of Health policies are only applicable down to the regional level. It is up to the local government units to adopt and adapt the policies to their own areas of jurisdiction.

The implementation of these guidelines and the monitoring of services demonstrate the huge gap between policy and reality. The Department of Health admits that it lacks a monitoring team or any system to ensure proper implementation of the hospital based-crisis centres. There have been reports that some hospitals do not comply with administrative order AO No. 1-Bs, even if they claim to have a women's desk. In 2001, only 14 of the reported 44 WCPUs submitted an annual report to the Department of Health.

1.1 Clinical management

In the clinical management of persons who have experienced sexual violence, the Department of Health adopts the Philippine General Hospital-Child Protection Unit and the Philippine General Hospital-Women's Desk protocols, which are not specific to sexual violence but to violence against women and children in general. The Department of Health respondent stated that the same protocols apply to men theoretically; however, most WCPUs have encountered no or very few male clients. While there is an expectation that such protocols may address men's needs, such a consideration was not taken into account by the authors of the protocols, which address forensic examination, short-term health care and psychological counselling, as well as long-term health care. Their use is included in the training that the Philippine General Hospital-Child Protection Unit and the Philippine General Hospital-Women's Desk conduct for WCPU doctors and nurses.

According to the Department of Health, for both women and men, only a gynaecologist with forensic training is authorized to conduct forensic examination. For child victims, the examination should be performed by a paediatrician with forensic training. They follow the protocol of the Philippine General Hospital–Child Protection Unit, as presented below.

For adult women patients, the Department of Health WCPUs are supposed to follow the protocol developed by the Philippine General Hospital-Women's Desk.

CHILD PROTECTION UNIT – PHILIPPINE GENERAL HOSPITAL
Overview of patient care

PATIENT INTAKE

- Patient and guardian greeted by CPU receptionist.
- Guardian completes consent form.
- Physician and social worker interview caretaker.
- Nurse plays with child in playroom.

FORENSIC INTERVIEW

- Physician conducts forensic interview that is both child-friendly and non-traumatizing, and is in adherence with legal guidelines for collecting evidence.
- Social worker listens to interview behind one-way mirror and takes notes. Social worker transcribes interview when necessary.
- Interviews may also be recorded by a video camera located on the other side of the one-way mirror. The video may then be presented in a court of law.

MEDICAL EXAMINATION

- Physician performs non-traumatizing medical examination that adheres to legal requirements for evidence collection, including colposcopic pictures.
- Physician also examines patient for medical problems not associated with abuse.
- Physician devises and implements a medical treatment plan.
- When necessary, referrals are made for medical services not provided by CPU, such as paediatric developmental assessment and other medical sub-specialties
- Medicine, food, clothes and transportation provided as needed.

RISK ASSESSMENT

- Social worker and physician conduct risk assessment for the child and family and decide on a plan of action that best protects the child and his or her family.
- Social worker takes steps to implement the action plan, such as placing the child in a shelter or having the perpetrator apprehended.
- Social worker and physician provide crisis counselling.

HOME VISIT
- Social worker conducts a home visit to all Metro Manila patients to assess the situation of the child and his or her family.
- Social worker conducts a second risk assessment and makes appropriate changes to the child's care plan

PSYCHIATRIC CARE
- Physician refers a patient who requires counselling to the psychiatrist.
- Psychiatrist conducts initial psychiatric screening and devises a treatment plan for the patient.
- Psychiatrist conducts regular therapy sessions for the child until the child shows significant improvement in his or her diagnosis.

CASE CONFERENCE
- Physician, psychiatrist and social worker conduct a weekly case conference about the patient's progress in psychotherapy.
- Physician and social worker conduct a case conference to discuss the child's progress after each home visit.
- Physician and social worker conduct case conferences with NGOs and government agencies to discuss CPU-endorsed cases.

REINTEGRATION
- Social worker works with patient and other involved agencies to reintegrate the child with his or her family, in a permanent shelter or with an adoptive family.

COURT TESTIMONY
- When summoned, CPU physicians appear in court to provide expert testimony about their findings.

GENDER-BASED VIOLENCE IN THE WESTERN PACIFIC REGION: A HIDDEN EPIDEMIC

GENERAL ALGORITHM FOR THE MANAGEMENT OF CASES OF VIOLENCE AGAINST WOMEN

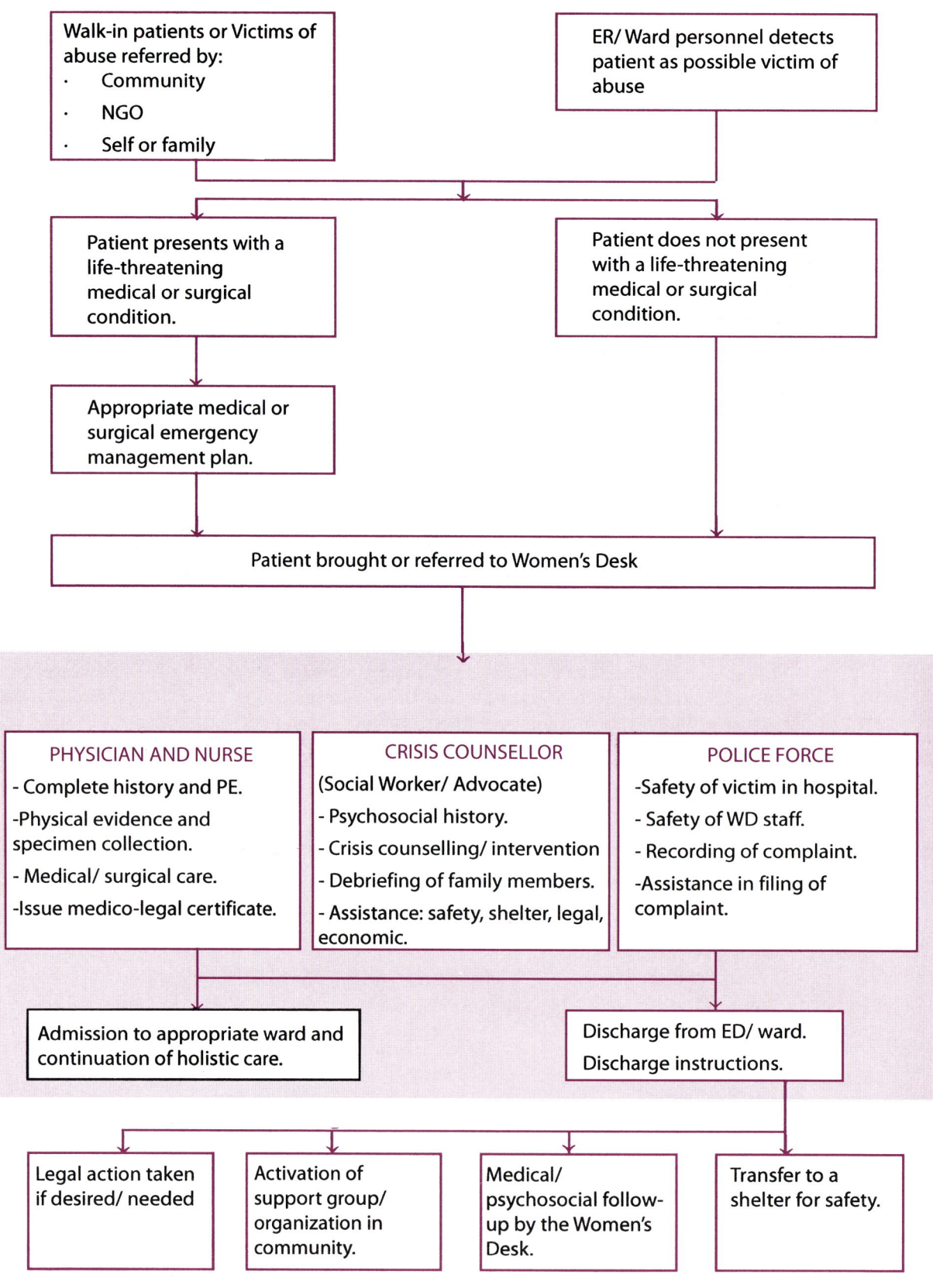

1.2 Training for forensic examiners

As mentioned, the Department of Health has an existing partnership with the Child Protection Unit of the Philippine General Hospital in training government health workers to provide health/medico-legal services to child victims of sexual violence. The memorandum of agreement between the two institutions, which was signed in 1999, states that the Child Protection Unit will train Department of Health physicians around the country to become child protection specialists. One paediatrician and one obstetrician–gynaecologist from each of the 16 regions of the Philippines undergo a six-week inservice training course at the Philippine General Hospital. The training sessions are cofunded by the Department of Health and the Advisory Board Foundation. To date, a total of 25 physicians have completed the training programme successfully.

Health professionals – physicians and nurses with forensic training, gynaecologists, emergency room doctors and nurses, and general practitioners - also undergo training on gender-based violence. The Department of Health collaborates with the Philippine General Hospital Women's Desk for the delivery of their inservice training on gender-based violence and medical management. Some hospitals also initiate gender-sensitivity training for their own staff. Some schools provide undergraduate training on gender-based violence and/or brief rotations in medico-legal institutions such as the Philippine National Police Crime Laboratory. An undergraduate curriculum on violence against women and children for nurses and doctors was piloted in Siliman University and Cebu Doctors College, and was launched in October 2000.

To ensure the continuation of the inservice training, and to monitor the implementation of the required services, the Department of Health hosts quarterly round-table discussions with the representatives of each WCPU. However, attendance at the quarterly meetings is sometimes less than satisfactory. As a result, the monitoring and updating of the status of most WCPUs is not optimal.

The Department of Health also has a 'Doctors to the *Barrios*' programme, whereby medical doctors are sent to far-flung areas to serve as municipal health officers. Prior to their deployment, the doctors receive training on various health concerns, including the handling of medico-legal cases. Training on providing medico-legal services is also given to the municipal health officers and hospital chiefs of staff of pilot provinces. It is a ten-day training seminar conducted by the Medico-legal Division of the National Bureau of Investigation.

The general objective of the medico-legal training is "to increase and update the technical knowledge, skills and abilities of the health officers of the local government units on legal medicine/forensic science, as well as to equip them with sufficient legal background to enable them to assist the courts in litigations regarding forensic expertise".

The course includes topics such as legal medicine; deception detection; use of polygraphs; medico-legal investigation and documentation; autopsy, deaths (including judicial deaths); physical injuries and trauma in general; asphyxia; forensic chemistry; firearm wounds; dactyloscopy; DNA collection, preparation and interpretation; medico-genital examination and sex crimes; crimes against persons; medical jurisprudence; court proceedings in medico-legal areas; and malpractice in general. The course ends with a mock court.

The topic of sex crimes (including medico-genital examination and DNA analysis) takes up one day of the ten-day training programme. Sub-topics include virginity and defloration; child abuse and situation; characteristics of child abuse; manifestations of victims of child abuse; and medico-legal examination of a victim of child abuse.

1.3 Equipment

When the WCPUs were established, 22 colposcopes were purchased and distributed all over the country. The physicians are trained by the Philippine General Hospital Child Protection

Unit on the use of this instrument. However, most of the colposcopes are now not working and their warranty periods have lapsed. While the hospitals are supposed to maintain the equipment, the respondent said that individual hospitals lack the funds to do so.

1.4 Attitudes

The Department of Health respondent believes that, aside from poverty, which is an indirect cause of sexual violence in society, the problem is also cultural – Filipino women are subservient, silent due to fear, and ignorant of their rights.

The Department of Health sees the health care workers' primary role in attending to a victim of sexual violence as providing psychosocial processing and counselling. The respondent believes that the victims come for solace. Physical assistance is secondary to psychological support. The respondent also believes that health care workers are advocates of women's health and rights in the prevention of sexual violence, a role which they fulfill through information campaigns.

The three main problems that the health sector faces in responding to cases of sexual violence are a lack of preparation or competency among health care workers; the inadequacy of networking at the local level, resulting in a lack of long-term assistance for the victims; and a lack of specific health facilities for survivors of abuse.

The Department of Health also sees a lack of attention and response given to the possibility of contracting sexually transmitted infections, especially HIV, as a result of sexual violence.

2. National Bureau of Investigation

The National Bureau of Investigation (NBI) is a centralized government agency providing investigative services for crimes, abuse, discrimination and exploitation. Alongside these services, the agency also provides technical services, such as forensic chemistry, neuropsychiatry and other medico-legal services. Although the main task of the NBI Medico-legal Division is examination of the victim and the gathering of evidence, it also offers first-aid treatment for injuries, whether or not evidence collection will be carried out. If a client requires more specialized management, he or she is referred to a hospital at this point. The Bureau also has a focal point for gender concerns, managed by a social worker who coordinates the provision of other services that a client may need, including shelter and counselling. However, in the written standard operating procedures, the provision of legal rights counselling or legal information is not mentioned.

2.1 Standard operating procedures in National Bureau of Investigation Headquarters

The NBI has its central office in the City of Manila and maintains four 'one-stop shops' and nine small clinics, with designated medical specialists, in various provinces (see Table 3). The funding for their operations comes from the national government.

Table 3. NBI medico-legal facilities

Facility	Luzon	Visayas	Mindanao
One-stop shops	National Capital Region (Manila) Tugeugarao-Isabela Baguio City, Mt. Province	Iloilo	Cagayan de Oro
Small clinics	La Union Pampanga Bicol Caraga	Cebu Leyte	Davao Cotabato Zamboanga

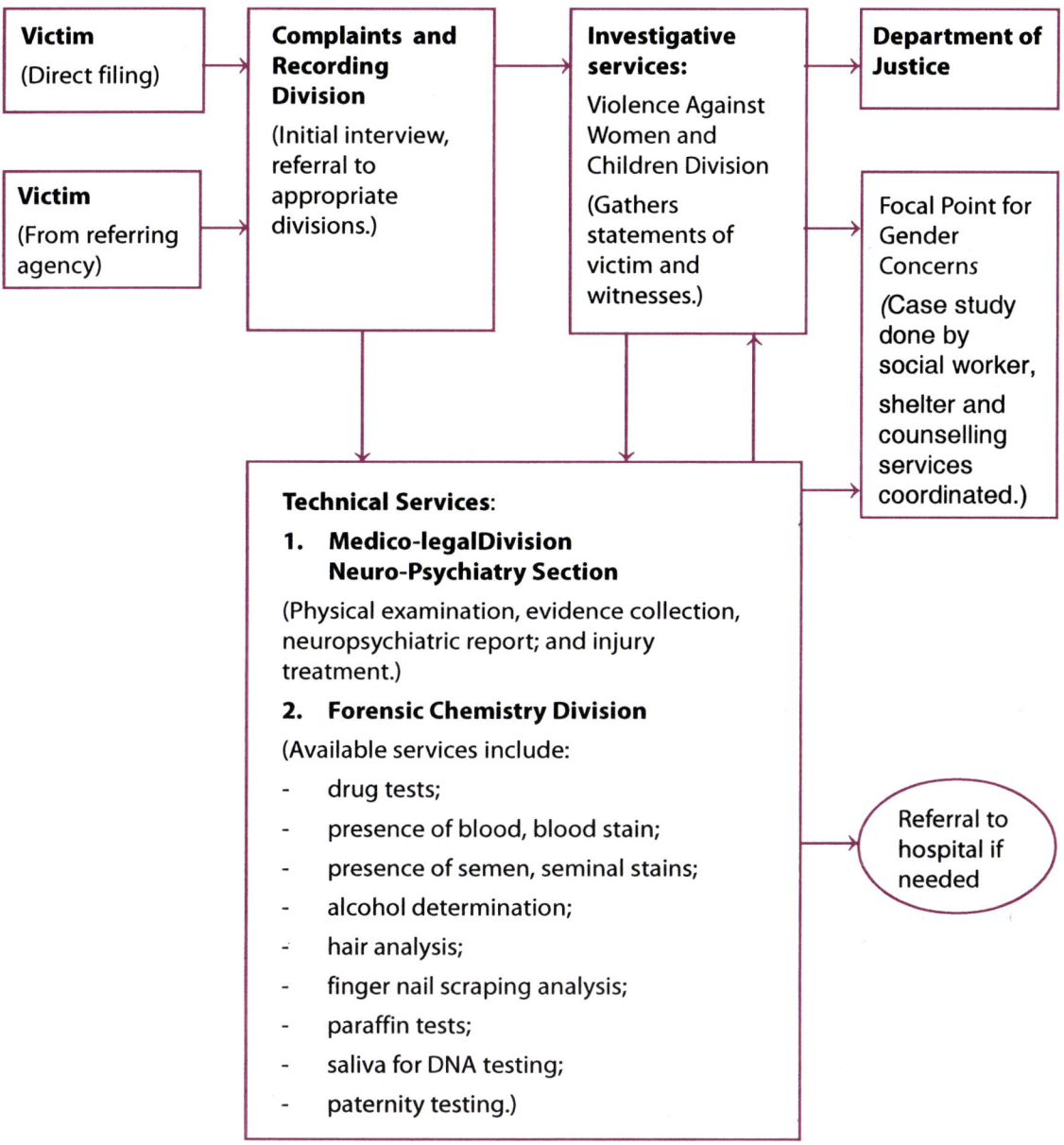

For those areas without one-stop shops or clinics, such as Region IV or Southern Tagalog Region, the NBI has a lone designated medico-legal officer (MLO) who handles the cases in all provinces of the region. These officers do not have adequate equipment and furnishings, and sometimes patients have to lie down on several chairs put together to be examined. The MLOs see female, child and male cases, although the latter is rare. To be able to receive medico-legal services from the NBI, a walk-in client has to obtain a written request from the NBI Regional Director's office or the police, who will issue a request for a medico-legal examination and forward that request to the MLO. Medico-legal examination may be conducted independent of a police report or intention to file a case. Initial treatment of injuries, on the other hand, is not provided in the regional office, since its task is limited to evidence collection

The medico-legal officer caries out a 'forensic examination' using the following steps:

(1) The MLO receives a request for forensic examination.

(2) The MLO conducts an interview and obtains consent for the procedures/ examination.

(3) The MLO conducts a medico-physico-genital examination.

(4) The MLO collects evidence.

(5) The MLO writes a report. For other health services that the client may require, he or she is referred to the hospital of choice.

2.2 Clinical management

Minimum procedures consist of physical and genital examinations, with the patient's consent (or parental consent for minors), and other ancillary laboratory services. If the client presents to the clinic within 72 hours of the sexual assault or rape, a vaginal smear for semen analysis will be performed automatically. A swab for possible DNA analysis is also taken. The respondent complained about the lack of storage facilities.

The smears are taken to the forensic laboratory in Manila by a registered nurse. Unfortunately, the unit lacks facilities for storing evidence. The chain of custody is also challenged frequently owing to the lack of protocol. In the regional office in Region IV, the forensic examiner himself delivers the specimens to the laboratory in Manila.

The Forensic Chemistry Division carries out semen analysis and gram staining as a matter of routine, but DNA analysis is deferred until the court orders it or the client requests it owing to the prohibitive price of the procedure (at least Php. 12000 or approximately US$ 240.00).

The NBI-Medico-legal Division at NBI Headquarters has no rape kits as defined. Instead, materials for taking vaginal smears for semen and DNA analysis are provided. What these consist of was not specified, however. The standard forensic examination, which basically consists of a physical examination and semen analysis, is offered free of charge. In Region IV, The NBI MLO prescribes the gloves and glass slides needed for the examination and smear test – the patients are thus expected to shoulder the costs of these materials themselves. The Division does not have any other equipment, such as a working colposcope, to aid its evidence collection.

The NBI-Medico-legal Division has a neuro-psychiatry section, and psychological testing and mental status examinations are carried out by a psychologist and a psychiatrist upon request. The results of these two separate tests are consolidated into one neuropsychiatric report.

For Region IV, the medico-legal office follows the same minimum procedure of securing consent for the medico-legal examination, history-taking, and 'medico-physico-genital examination'. The MLO notes any external injuries, signs of haematoma, lacerations and the appearance of the genitalia. A swab is taken if the patient comes in within 72 hours of the alleged attack. The examiner also conducts an internal examination. The office/ clinic is not equipped with a colposcope. Neither does it have a neuropsychiatry section, such as is found in NBI Headquarters. A report is written up by the MLO after the interview and the physico-genital examination.

2.3 Training

The NBI provides an inservice course on forensic examination for medical doctors and nurses who join the Medico-legal Division. The Bureau imposes no other special requirements/prior training on any related specialty for physicians who are admitted to the NBI, save for passing the medical licensure examination given by the Professional Regulation Commission. The training lasts between three to six months for doctors and is handled by the Medico-legal Division. The training programme consists of hands-on training on performing medico-legal examinations, autopsy, preparing appropriate reports, and mock courts. There is no mechanism in place to monitor the adequacy of the training. Nor is there an accreditation system for forensic examiners, except for a *revalida* (revalidation) examination given at the end of the training. After passing that examination, the medical doctor gains the title 'Medico-legal Officer' and may then be assigned to any NBI office in the country. There are no mechanisms in place to ensure the continuation of inservice training, and the trainees are not given any incentives to attend such training. Promotion is largely based on the length of service rendered in the institution. The title of 'Medico-legal Officer II' may be awarded after two to three years.

The health professionals in the Medico-legal Division, such as the doctors and nurses with forensic training, also undergo training on gender-based violence, sponsored by either nongovernmental organizations or the Bureau itself. The training involves a three-day inservice session with the objective of increasing awareness and sensitivity to gender-based issues.

2.4 Policies

The NBI follows RA 8505 – the Rape Victims' Assistance Act, which requires female victims to be seen by female doctors. In the absence of a female doctor, the victim may be examined by a male physician provided that a chaperone is present. In the NBI, there are four female physicians and five male. The former are assigned to examine clients in the clinic while the latter are assigned to autopsies.

The NBI respondent was unaware if there are mechanisms in place to disseminate their policies to health care professionals.

2.5 Attitudes

The respondent from NBI Headquarters believes that one of the causes of sexual violence in the country is poverty. Poor economic conditions force people to share rooms and restrooms. As a result, sexual violence is easily perpetrated against vulnerable individuals. The high level of overseas employment means that many children are left without adequate protection, especially from the mother, making them more vulnerable to incest. Drugs and alcohol also influence the commission of sexual violence. The MLO from Region IV holds the same views and added pornography to the list of causes of sexual violence in the country.

The NBI respondent said that the NBI's role is not the prevention of sexual violence *per se*, but the management of victims. The NBI does not initiate campaigns against sexual violence. However, the respondent from Region IV believes that the flow of illicit drugs should be stopped first if the problem of sexual abuse if to be solved.

As for the NBI, non-reporting of cases by victims is seen as the main problem faced by the institution in providing medico-legal services to those who need them.

The NBI would like to raise the issue of lack of reagents for laboratory screening for sexually transmitted diseases among victims. Likewise, there is no funding for advocacy campaigns against sexual violence. The Bureau would also like to strengthen the follow up of cases by social workers.

3. The Philippine National Police

There are two pathways by which a victim of sexual violence can access medico-legal services from the Philippine National Police. The first is through the Women's and Children's Desks located at local police stations, and the second is through the Women's Crisis and Child Protection Center, located at Philippine National Police Headquarters.

An overview of the development of medico-legal services for female and child victims of sexual violence is presented below, culled from the official website of the Philippine National Police (PNP):

Addressing women's and children's concerns has been given priority in the area of law enforcement and community relations by the Philippine National Police since the National Police Commission issued Memorandum Circular Number 92-010, which paved the way for the establishment of the Child and Youth Relations Section (CYRS) in highly urbanized cities, including Metro Manila, and the designation of Child and Youth Relations Officers in other police stations nationwide.

Awareness of the alarming number of cases of victimization of children and young women due to sexual exploitation resulted in the enactment of RA 7610 (Special Protection of Children Against Child Abuse, Exploitation and Discrimination Act) on 17 June 1992. The PNP forged a working partnership with other concerned government agencies, particularly the Social Welfare and Justice Departments, as well as nongovernmental organizations, to raise the consciousness of the police force about the rights of women and children and the necessary police intervention for the protection of those rights, especially from exploitation, harm and danger.

Soon came the establishment, in 1993, of the first Women's Desk in Quezon City, a project of the Directorate for Police Community Relations and the National Commission on the Role of Filipino Women, with NGO participation. That project was replicated in other major cities and spread like wildfire across other parts of the country even before RA 8551, otherwise known as the PNP Reform and Reorganization Act of 1998, was enacted. Title VII of the law amplified the institutionalization of the Management of Cases of Children in Especially Difficult Circumstances, which contains certain procedures in the handling of children's cases. It was published in 1992. The PNP Directorate for Investigation and Detective Management has also published the *PNP Handbook on Child Abuse and Neglect*, which deals with child interview techniques and the dynamics of child sexual abuse and its medico-legal implications, of which the police should also be aware.

In June 1997, the Women's Desk and the Child and Youth Relations Section (CYRS) were merged into one, now the Women and Children's Desk, in order to strengthen and optimize the use of policewomen in responding to cases and concerns of women and children. The structural make-up of the Women and Children's Desk was formalized by the activation of the Women and Children Concerns Division (WCCD) under the Directorate for Police Community Relations (DPCR), following the issuance of PNP Memorandum Circular Number 97-001, dated September 1997.

The WCCD has since been an effective component of the PNP, exercising supervision, monitoring and evaluation; providing policy direction; and formulating programmes and projects geared towards the effective operation of the Women' and Children's Desks. In January 1998, the PNP adopted a data monitoring system for cases involving women and children victims of abuse and violence with a view to establishing a profile of all such cases that would subsequently serve as basis for PNP policy and programme formulation for women and children.

Women and children victim-survivors of sexual violence who come to the local police stations for assistance (especially those outside Metro Manila) are attended to by the local Women and Children's Desk and may be referred to their hospital of choice or the nearest PNP crime laboratory for medico-legal examination. The crime laboratories are located in the PNP Headquarters, eight technical divisions, five NCR district offices, 15 regional offices, and several provincial and city field offices. The functions of the crime laboratories include conducting forensic examinations on all physical evidences such as:

- medico-legal examination;
- forensic examination;

- forensic document analysis;
- forensic personal identification through dactyloscopy of fingerprint examination and identification;
- ballistics examination and identification;
- forensic photography;
- polygraph or lie detection test;
- composite criminal illustration;
- scene of crime processing on operation (SOCO); and
- DNA examination (future capability)

In 2000, there were 1490 Women and Children's Desks situated at 95% of all police stations nationwide. In 2003, responsibility for the Women and Children's Desks was transferred to the Directorate for Investigation and Detective Management.

The other medico-legal facility within the police force is the Women's Crisis and Child Protection Center (WCCPC), which was activated in January 2001 at the PNP National Headquarters in Camp Crame, under the Directorate for Police Community Relations. Its vision is to "investigate, safeguard, assist and provide multi-disciplinary treatment to women and children victims of abuse and violence…with the end in view of helping ensure the victim's rehabilitation, recovery and reintegration into the community and of serving the ends of justice." The composite team is composed of police professionals from the Criminal Investigation and Detection Group, the Crime Laboratory and Health Services. The project was jointly initiated by the PNP, the Philippine General Hospital, and the Advisory Board Foundation, a Washington-based NGO which is working closely with the Philippine General Hospital in the area of child abuse treatment. The Royal Netherlands Embassy in the Philippines and the United Nations Children's Fund (UNICEF) have provided some equipment necessary for its operation.

Services offered in the WCCPC include:

- appropriate police investigation of all cases involving violence against women and children;
- highest standards of medico-legal, psychological/ psychiatric and counselling services to female and child victims of violence;
- collection and preservation of evidence for use in the prosecution of cases of violence against women and children;
- prevention of retraumatization of female and child victims of violence by providing them optimum professional care and attention;
- assistance in providing intervention to female and child victims of violence for their rehabilitation, recovery and subsequent reintegration into the community;
- coordination with other agencies concerned with the protection of women and children;
- filing of cases of violence against women and children with the courts; and
- tracking and follow-up of cases

PNP Circular Number 2001-002, dated January 16 2001, specifies that procedures for cases of violence against women and children referred by the local police to Camp Crame for medico-legal examination will be as follows:

- If sexual/ physical abuse against children – refer to WCCPC.
- If sexual abuse against women – refer to WCCPC.
- If other forms of abuse/ crimes against women – refer to the Crime Laboratory.

In 2003, responsibility for the WCCPC was transferred to the Directorate for Investigation and Detective Management.

Subsequent discussions on management, training, equipment and attitudes will be largely based on the experience of the PNP WCCPC at the National Headquarters in Camp Crame.

3.1 Clinical management

According to the PNP respondents, most victims usually go first to their *barangay* office since most victims do not know the proper steps to follow. The *barangay* officer directs them to the proper channels. However, most of the clients at the PNP WCCPC/Crime Laboratory Headquarters are referred by the police, the Women's Crisis Center, the Department of Social Welfare and Development, *Bantay Bata* or directly from *barangay*s. The choice of facility accessed by victims depends on the specialty of the services offered or their proximity. In the twelve months preceding this study, the WCCPC saw around 200 patients, averaging around 1-5 patients per day. The facility is open on weekdays only, from 8:00 am to 5:00 pm.

The WCCPC physicians consider a person who has suffered sexual violence to be a serious medical case. This, to them, is the reason why the rape crisis centres are located very close to the emergency rooms of hospitals. Thus, they provide health care independent of forensic examination. A police report is not a requirement for receiving a medico-legal examination. These services are performed free of charge.

Although the WCCPC is housed in the PNP General Hospital, its clients cannot access the medical services of that hospital since it is exclusive to members of the PNP and their dependents. There are instances when the medico-legal officers have to transfer clients to the East Avenue Medical Center (or the client's hospital of choice) for tertiary-level treatment. In such cases, the MLO accompanies the patient to the hospital so he can perform the forensic examination simultaneously with health care management. Chaperones are also available during the forensic or medical examinations. Those who can act as chaperones include sexual violence care advocates (CPU nurses, doctors, investigators), social workers, mental health care practitioners, police personnel, and relatives or friends of the client.

Informed consent is always secured prior to forensic examination. In getting the consent, the step-by-step procedure is disclosed to the client. According to the respondent, the current standard operating procedure for forensic examination of acute cases is to "first obtain a swab then test for the presence of spermatozoa. The cotton applicator sticks are sent to the DNA laboratory where they are stored and examined/analysed only after a court order." The Crime Laboratory used to have a free supply of the acid phosphatase reagent from the Federal Bureau of Investigation. It was used to determine the presence of spermatozoa, a test routinely done for acute cases (within 72 hours of sexual assault).

The forensic evidence is labelled and signed by the doctor, with the date and time. It is placed in a filing cabinet that is locked and only opened subsequently upon court order. An evidence custodian is in charge of storage. The clients' records are also kept in a locked filing cabinet, to which even doctors have limited access.

Although the medico-legal examiners regularly raise the issue of HIV with their clients, no further services are provided. The respondents claim that they lack training regarding counselling on HIV and they do not have an institution to which to refer patients. As for testing for other STIs, the physicians get a sample of vaginal/penile discharge and make a request for laboratory examination for gonorrhoea, chlamydia or trichomonas. It is up to the client to take the specimens to their laboratory of choice, as this service is not available in the facility. Sexually transmitted infection prophylaxis is provided regularly. Treatment plans are developed for medical follow-up of victims, especially for those who have contracted STIs.

The issue of pregnancy is also raised regularly with female victims. The physicians ask about and discuss contraceptive use, and conduct pregnancy testing if necessary. They offer emergency contraception, "even if the Department of Health Secretary is against it."

Assessment of the victim's psychological state is also one of the services provided. Counselling is provided, although more difficult cases are referred to the National Center for Mental Health, the Women's Crisis Center or a feminist counsellor.

Clients are regularly referred to the police, legal aid (such as the Women's Legal Bureau, the Women's League, the Integrated Bar of the Philippines) or social services for any pertinent assistance they may need. They are given information on the services available, the follow-up required and the community resources available. The information is printed in brochures which are distributed at the PNP Women's Desks.

The PNP MLOs give evidence/ expert testimony in court frequently, attending an average of 8-15 court hearings per month. The problems they encounter include frequent postponement of hearings due to absence of fiscals, and a lack of transportation to the various regional trial courts. The respondents lamented that there are fiscals (prosecutors) who do not know how to ask questions of medico-legal expert witnesses. For example, there are lawyers who ask if the patient was raped. The MLOs have to explain that physicians do not make a diagnosis of rape; that determination is up to the court.

The respondent further stressed that the medico-legal examination will only corroborate the disclosure of a victim. As such, it is dispensable. Therefore, the respondent maintained that the one important 'tool' is the victim's testimony.

3.2 Equipment

A working colposcope, donated by the Advisory Board Foundation, is available at the PNP WCCPC for examination and documentation. Although there are no rape kits available for collecting evidence, the WCCPC has a supply of cotton swabs, manila envelopes and paper bags. They collect articles of clothing, which are air-dried and stored and preserved in envelopes or paper bags.

3.3 Policies and protocols

The WCCPC has adopted the policies and protocols of the Philippine General Hospital.

3.4 Training

The MLOs of the WCCPC undergo a one-year inservice course on medico-legal issues, including gender and sexual violence. The training is provided by the institution, as well as by nongovernmental organizations such as the Women's Crisis Center, the Lunduyan Foundation and UNICEF. The Philippine General Hospital Child Protecion Unit also conducts training on child protection. The WCCPC also provides lectures and training sessions to other organizations on these matters.

3.5 Attitudes

The health care providers from the PNP-Crime Laboratory see sexual violence as a health problem, a criminal justice problem, a social problem and a psychosocial problem. They consider a person who has suffered sexual violence to be a serious medical case – citing this view as the logic behind building the rape crisis centres (or women and child protection units) very near the emergency rooms in most hospitals with such facilities. Moreover, they believe that, aside from providing medical care, they are also advocates, fulfilling that role by providing lectures to health and NGO workers on sexual violence issues.

3.6 First points of entry into the formal assistance system

According to the macro-level respondents from the Department of Health and the NBI, the possible first points of entry into the formal assistance system for men, women and children are:

- the NBI;

- government-designated health centres for victims of violence, tertiary and regional hospitals; or

- police facilities for victims of violence, such as the Crime Laboratory of the Philippine National Police.

They may also go directly to police stations and the court (i.e., fiscal's office). However, from the PNP's experience, most victims do not know the proper steps to follow and they often approach their *barangay* office (village council) first to ask where they should go next.

In contrast, according to the micro-level respondents of the survey (i.e., service providers and client proxies), the initial points of entry chosen by victims of sexual attacks are the police (22 out of 68), social workers (21 out of 68) and medico-legal-facilities (11 out of 68). Other first points of entry indicated by the micro-level respondents included: rural health units, *barangay* offices and nearest hospitals. Table 5 shows, by type of respondent, the top five entry-points accessed by victims of sexual violence.

Most victims, in the opinion of the macro-level respondents, go to government-run designated health centres because of their low income status. However, it should be noted that one limitation of this study is that only government hospitals were sampled. The behaviour of victims of higher socioeconomic status cannot, therefore, be adequately described, since most of them go to private hospitals.

The availability of specialized services or designated health centres for victims of sexual violence in hospitals retained by the Department of Health, such as regional hospitals, also determines the type of facility accessed. Proximity is another substantial factor in the choice of facility approached. If a victim wishes to register a case, she or he will most often go to the medico-legal offices or police facilities for victims of violence.

All respondents claimed that the same services and processes apply to men, women and children alike. They noted, however, that they rarely encounter male complainants.

As for Region IV, the NBI MLO stated that most victims go to district hospitals or private hospitals first for medical treatment. They may also approach the Department of Social Welfare and Development for assistance. However, if a victim wishes to register a case, she approaches the NBI office in her region or goes directly to the PNP Crime Laboratory in Manila. The NBI MLOs also often advise clients to go directly to the NBI Headquarters in Manila, arguing that the services there are more complete. (The provinces in the Southern Tagalog Region, except the islands of Palawan, Romblon and Mindoro and Marinduque, are only a few hours away from Metro Manila by land transportation). The choice of facilities approached by clients largely depends on their proximity.

Table 5 lists the top three factors determining the entry-point into the formal assistance system according to micro-level respondents:

These results conform to the criteria used by victims to decide where to go initially after a sexual attack, as identified by the respondents on the victims' behalf. The number of service providers and client proxies (24 out of 67) who answered 'specialty of service' as a basis for choosing first points of entry is comparable with those who indicated 'legal requirements for a sexual violence case' (23 out of 67). Other responses included: 'availability of medical doctors', and 'approachability' of the staff.

MICRO LEVEL

1. Types of facilities surveyed

Of the eight health facilities surveyed, three were tertiary hospitals, three district hospitals, one a secondary hospital and one a designated health centre for victims of sexual violence. The funding source for these facilities is the national, provincial, or city government, as they are all public in nature. Some facility managers said that they were also receiving fiscal support from donor and insurance agencies, while one of them indicated providing out-of-pocket funds.

It should be stressed that the health facilities sampled for the micro-level study are not under the Department of Health, since the health system has been devolved to the local government units, starting from the provincial level down to the small village health stations.

According to the service managers, all the facilities sampled offer acute health care. Four of them claim that they offer forensic examination services (i.e. evidence collection and analysis) and one, long-term health care (i.e. psychological counselling) to victims of sexual assault. However, it is clear that forensic services are not provided for in half of the facilities sampled. Also, the data reveal that health care for sexual violence cases is not being given much attention, as represented by the non-specialized and short-term service provision being offered to victims.

Table 4. Services offered according to facility managers (n = 8)

Types of service	YES	NO	OTHERS*
HIV testing	2	5	1
HIV counselling	4	3	1
Antiretrovirals (drug therapy for AIDS)	2	5	1
Counselling on pregnancy	6	1	1
Emergency contraception	1	6	1
Abortion counselling	2	5	1
STI screening	4	3	1
STI treatment	4	2	2
Counselling	5	1	2
Referrals to other sectors	7	0	1

* Response includes *don't know* and *no reply*

There is no common protocol and therefore no consciousness of having to meet minimum procedural requirements. This is clearly reflected by the types of services being provided, according to facility managers. Only half of those interviewed routinely provide STI screening and HIV testing.

2. Where victims go first and why

Table 5. First points of entry for sexual violence victims, by respondent type

First Points of Entry	Medical doctors	Forensic examiners	Registered nurses	Client proxies	% (over n=68)
Police	5	2	3	12	41.2%
Social worker	3	0	3	15	30.9%
Medico-legal facility (i.e. NBI)	0	1	6	4	16.2%
Police facility (i.e. PNP Women's Desk)	2	1	2	2	10.3%
District hospital	3	0	1	2	8.8%

According to the service providers and client proxies, the initial points of entry chosen by victims of sexual attacks are the police (22 out of 68), social workers (21 out of 68) and medico-legal facilities (11 out of 68). Other first points of entry indicated by the respondents include: rural health units, *barangay* offices and nearest hospitals.

These results conform to the criteria used by victims to decide where to go initially after a sexual attack, as identified by the respondents on the victims' behalf. The number of service providers and client proxies (24 out of 67) who answered 'specialty of service' as a basis for choosing first points of entry is comparable with those who indicated 'legal requirements for a sexual violence case' (23 out of 67). The results, however, do not indicate that those who considered legal requirements as a criterion for selection actually file cases against their attackers. Other responses include: 'availability of medical doctors', and 'approachability' of staff.

Table 6. Criteria for selecting first points of entry

Criteria	% (over n=67)
Specialty of the service (health, forensic, etc.)	35.8%
Legal requirements for a sexual violence case	34.3%
Proximity	28.4%

3. Process

Table 7. Persons who escort victims to the service facility

Persons escorting victims	% (over n=68)
Family	88.2%
Social welfare representatives	47.1%
Friends	45.6%
On their own	27.9%
Police	23.5%

A total of 60 out of the 68 respondents (88.2%) indicated family members as the key persons who accompany sexual violence victims to service facilities. Other persons who escort the victims include teachers and *barangay* officials. About 60% (40 out of 68) claimed that victims come to their facility before going to the police, which may lend explanation to the lower response rate regarding police representatives as companions of victims seeking health care assistance.

Among the 37 health practitioners interviewed, 32 (86.5%) do not require a police report before administering medical examinations and 36 (97.3%) claim that sexual violence victims are attended to clinically free of charge.

The study revealed that the waiting time before a victim of sexual violence is given medical attention ranges from 0-4 hours, depending on the availability of the examining physician. Approximately 25% of the service providers replied that victims wait for about 5 minutes (9 out of 37) to 30 minutes (9 out of 34), on average, before being examined.

Only 21.6% (8 out of 37) of the service providers require informed consent from the victim before administering medical examinations. The remaining 78.4% either do not demand written consent forms or made no reply to the question. It is alarming that only a small minority are conscious of the need to secure informed consent from victims, whether verbal or written. Some responses indicate a misconception that consent is implied upon the victim's presentation to a facility, whereas informed consent, in the strict sense, requires that the procedures to be undertaken are fully understood and accepted by the client.

4. Content of care

The data show that more than half of the health care providers raise issues which are of significant concern to sexually abused persons. Of the 37 health care professionals, 51.4% said they regularly raise the issue of HIV/AIDS, 61.1% (22 of 36) raise the issue of pregnancy with female victims, and 56.8% (21 of 37) raise the issue of STIs with victims of sexual violence. The health services rendered to victims by physicians and nurses are summarized in Table 8.

Table 8. Medical care provided by health practitioners (over n=37)

Type of medical care	%YES	%NO	%OTHERS*
HIV and related issues	51.4	29.7	18.9
Offer HIV counselling	27.0	29.7	43.2
Offer HIV testing	10.8	45.9	43.2
Advise client where to go for HIV test	32.4	24.3	43.2
Offer antiretrovirals	00.0	56.8	43.2
Pregnancy and related issues**	61.1	25.0	13.9
Ask about and discuss contraceptive use	16.2	59.5	24.3
Discuss pregnancy testing	56.8	18.9	24.3
Offer emergency contraceptives	2.70	73.0	24.3
Provide abortion counselling	2.70	73.0	24.3
STI and related issues	56.8	32.4	10.8
STI screening	37.8	48.6	13.5
STI prophylaxis	5.4	81.1	13.5
Referral for STI treatment	29.7	56.8	13.5

* Response included *don't know* and *no reply*
** n = 36

A little more than half of the respondents claimed to raise the issue of HIV, pregnancy and STI. However, on further questioning, very few said they provide specific services such as counselling, testing and other long-term follow-up services. At present, the respondents seem to have no consensus on giving rape victims emergency contraception options, because official Department of Health policy prohibits their use. Some service providers have resorted to prescribing high-dose estrogen-progesterone preparations as an emergency contraceptive measure.

The results suggest that the service staff are conscious about the more sensitive health issues vis-à-vis sexual violence. However, the lack of drugs, reagents, referral information and other essential resources is impeding the delivery of those services. Regarding pregnancy, the figures clearly reflect the religious leaning of the respondents (i.e. against contraceptive use and abortion).

The majority of the service providers (almost 75%) assess the psychological state of victims, and nearly 65% (24 of 37) provide counselling, indicating that they are indeed sensitive to the psychosocial dimensions of sexual violence. Furthermore, about 81% (30 of 37 respondents) refer victims to other sectors, particularly to social services and mental health professionals. For assistance in other matters, victims are referred to the NBI, NGOs, Camp Crame, or PNP Women's Desks.

Of the 37 respondents, 20 (54.1%) said that they provide information and support to sexual violence victims on the procedures followed, required follow-up and available community resources, while 19 (51.4%) do not regularly develop a treatment plan for medical follow-up of sexual violence victims. It should be noted that over half of the providers seem concerned with providing necessary information to victims. However, despite the providers' concerns over the psychological state of victims, non-participation in the development of a treatment plan may indicate they are not as active in the rehabilitation process of the victims.

5. Equipment

Table 9 shows that the supply of equipment and other items related to health service delivery for sexually-abused persons is limited. Only two facilities possess a 'rape kit', the medico-legal service facility in the capital and a provincial tertiary hospital. Inexpensive items essential for evidence collection, such as combs, tweezers, paper sheets and paper bags, are also generally lacking. Drugs for the treatment of STIs, antiretrovirals and emergency contraceptives are available in fewer than half of the facilities sampled for the study, and service managers noted that such drugs are in short supply. Such data have significant implications for the quality and extent of health assistance that can be provided to victims of sexual violence.

Table 9. Percentage (%) of facilities possessing item, by study site

Items	Capital city (n=3)	Provinces (n=5)	TOTAL (n=8)
Equipment:			
1. Magnifying glass (or colposcope)	25.0	25.0	50.0
2. Access to an autoclave to sterilize equipment	37.5	62.5	100.0
3. Microscope	37.5	62.5	100.0
4. 'Rape kit' for collection of forensic evidence	12.5	12.5	25.0
5. Speculum	37.5	62.5	100.0
6. Comb for collecting foreign matter in pubic hair	12.5	25.0	37.5
7. Syringes and needles	37.5	62.5	100.0
8. Tubes for collecting blood	37.5	62.5	100.0
9. Glass slides for preparing wet and/or dry mounts (for sperm)	37.5	62.5	100.0
10. Swabs for collecting samples	37.5	62.5	100.0
11. Laboratory containers for transporting swabs	25.0	50.0	75.0
12. Urine specimen containers	37.5	62.5	100.0
13. Toludine blue solution (1%) as colourant, and acetic acid (1%) as decolourant	12.5	37.5	50.0
14. Tweezers/ scissors for collecting foreign debris on skin	12.5	50.0	72.5
15. Paper sheet for collecting debris as the survivor undresses	12.5	25.0	37.5
16. Tape measure for measuring the size of bruises, lacerations, etc.	37.5	62.5	100.0
17. Paper bags for collection of evidence	12.5	25.0	37.5
18. Supplies for universal precautions from contamination	0.0	12.5	12.5
19. Resuscitation equipment for anaphylactic reactions	25.0	50.0	75.0
20. Sterile medical instruments (kit) and suture material for repair of tears	25.0	62.5	87.5
21. Spare items of clothing to replace those that are torn or taken for evidence	12.5	12.5	25.0
22. Sanitary supplies (pads or local cloths)	12.5	62.5	75.0
23. Gauzes and other wound treatment supplies	37.5	62.5	100.0
24. Pregnancy tests	37.5	62.5	100.0
25. Pregnancy calculator disk to determine the age of a pregnancy	25.0	50.0	75.0
26. Examination gloves	37.5	62.5	100.0
Drugs:			
27. For treatment of STIs (doxycycline, clindamycin))	25.0	25.0	50.0
28. Antiretrovirals (acyclovin)	12.5	0.0	12.5
29. Emergency contraception (pills, i.e. Depo-provera®)	25.0	12.5	37.5
30. Tetanus toxoid, tetanus immunoglobulin	25.0	50.0	75.0
31. Hepatitis B vaccine	25.0	25.0	50.0
32. Pain relief (e.g. paracetamol)	37.5	50.0	87.5
33. Anxiolytic (e.g. diazepam)	25.0	37.5	62.5
34. Sedative for children (e.g. diazepam)	25.0	25.0	50.0
35. Local anaesthetic for suturing	25.0	62.5	87.5
36. Antibiotics for wound care	37.5	50.0	87.5
Administrative supplies:			
37. Medical chart with pictograms	37.5	37.5	75.0
38. Forms for recording post-rape care	0.0	50.0	50.0
39. Consent forms	37.5	62.5	100.0
40. Information pamphlets for post-rape care (for survivor)	12.5	12.5	25.0
41. List of names and addresses of referral sites	25.0	50.0	75.0
42. Surveillance forms to record basic data about client cases	12.5	37.5	50.0
43. Computer to manage client information and facility statistics	12.5	25.0	37.5
44. Refrigerator/ freezer to store forensic evidence	12.5	37.5	50.0
45. Safe, locked filing space to keep confidential records	12.5	37.5	50.0

6. Policies and protocol

About 35.1% (13 of 37) of the service providers claimed that there is a policy that guides their work on sexual violence, while only 27% (10 of 37) use a service protocol in the provision of services for victims of sexual attacks. These figures do not seem to match the response of the facility managers, half of whom indicated that there is such a policy, while five out of the eight managers maintained the presence of a service protocol. The disagreement between the responses may be attributed to the lack of service staff training on the use of the aforementioned procedure, as well as the inefficient information dissemination processes.

7. Safety

Five of the eight facility managers reported that incidences of violence had been registered within their service facilities. However, half of them signified a lack of standard procedures to respond to such occurrences. Furthermore, according to five of the respondents, safety mechanisms against violent incidents seem to be deficient.

Table 10. Availability of safety measures, by study site

Safety measures	Capital city (n=3)	Provinces (n=5)	TOTAL (n=8)
1. Guards	25.0	62.5	87.5
2. Alarms	25.0	25.0	50.0
3. Portable phones	25.0	50.0	75.0
4. Restricted public access	25.0	37.5	62.5
5. Separation of victim and perpetrator in waiting area	25.0	50.0	75.0
6. Separation of victim and perpetrator in examination area	25.0	50.0	75.0

It should be noted that none of the facilities sampled for the study are completely equipped with the safety measures indicated in Table 10. It also seems that victims are not guaranteed safety from perpetrators, either in the waiting or the examination areas. Such conditions may put more stress on victims and may hinder the treatment process.

8. Attitudes

Table 11. Categorization of sexual violence, by respondent type

Category	Medical doctors	Forensic examiners	Registered nurses	Client proxies	% (over n=68)
Social problem	15	2	16	27	88.2%
Criminal justice problem	13	2	17	25	83.8%
Health problem	9	1	15	15	58.8%

It is interesting to note that more health service providers regard sexual violence as a social and criminal justice problem than a health problem. Such views certainly have implications for health service delivery, as health care provision may not be deemed by those providers to be a primary response to sexual violence cases. In addition, one nurse said she perceives sexual violence as a 'family problem'.

9. Training

More than 75% (28 out of 37) of the health practitioners had received no training on sexual violence. The rest responded that they had received relevant training of the following types: post-graduate courses, inservice training, cross-project visits and seminars. According to them, the topics covered in the courses included, among others: human sexuality, psychosocial aspects of sexual violence, counselling and referral procedures. Health providers from the local government units acknowledged a major lack of training on sexual violence, particularly on forensic services, such as evidence collection and documentation, as well as on issues concerning the criminal justice system.

10. Multisectoral collaboration

The majority of the respondents expressed satisfaction about the assistance provided by the judiciary, the police and the health sector. However, such comments do not translate into adequate performance of the aforementioned agencies in responding to matters concerning sexual violence.

Chapter 6.
DISCUSSION

STRENGTHS

While sensitive to the psychosocial consequences that sexual attacks can inflict on victims, most of the service providers do not develop treatment plans for patients.

The victims and their relatives are able to identify the agencies that may be of assistance to them when faced with circumstances pertaining to sexual violence, such as the police and health care facilities. The referral system regarding cases of sexual abuse, however, needs to be adequately defined and the role to be played by each sector has to be made clear to all stakeholders. It was observed that, on some occasions, there is unnecessary duplication in the services rendered by the police and the medico-legal facility. Such inefficiencies in service delivery certainly impose an undue burden and inconvenience on victims of sexual abuse.

QUALITY OF CARE

1. Improve health status

The present health service provision for sexual violence cases seems insufficient to improve the victims' health status significantly. There are several concerns that demand adequate attention, specifically matters related to resource availability. The lack of adequate materials and supplies is compromising the quality of health care that can be delivered to clients.

2. Ensure adequate documentation of evidence

The primary factor that was observed as hindering adequate evidence documentation is the delayed reporting of cases, several years for some victims. Under such circumstances, it is nearly impossible to collect useful data that can substantiate claims that an attack has occurred, especially taking into consideration the absence of equipment and the inability of most victims to access services that involve costly charges.

Another problem that has to be addressed is the need for provision of storage facilities to secure evidence. Because of the lack of such facilities, the chain of evidence is not guaranteed.

3. Ensure satisfaction of client expectations

It seems that victims, as well as their relatives, are not well informed about the procedures that should be followed. Because of this, they are also uncertain in their expectations with regard to the role the different agencies can play in the processing and management of their complaints.

4. Ensure involvement of community

From the study, it seems that community involvement begins and ends with the assistance of *barangay* representatives in the reporting of sexual violence cases. Moreover, in situations when perpetrators are related to victims, community members seem hesitant to involve themselves in the issue.

Chapter 7.
CONCLUSIONS

The majority of victims proceed to police stations, special police facilities and government social workers on matters concerning sexual violence. This suggests an overwhelming perception that sexual violence is primarily a criminal justice and social concern rather than a health issue. Therefore, if priorities are to be addressed, the study clearly indicates the need to further systematize and enhance capacities for therapeutic interventions among non-health sectors (i.e. police, social workers). Such efforts must highlight the fact that sexual violence has possible long-term health consequences and that it is not solely a criminal justice or social issue.

Considering that the entry points into the formal assistance system are at the local government level and that proximity is one of the major factors in utilization of facilities, there should be an effort to advocate and provide support for the training of local government unit service providers. It may be that the regional referral centres (WCPUs in regional hospitals) are insufficient to meet the needs of victims.

The huge involvement of family members as persons who escort victims to service facilities is confirmed by the study. This indicates the need to improve family education and management in any future medical protocols/ standards. However, the possibility that family members are also perpetrators should be considered, especially in cases of child sexual abuse. In such instances, child victims should be interviewed alone whenever possible. These ethical issues in the management of survivors need to be emphasized and addressed in the design of the protocols and training curriculum.

A positive point is that most of the service providers claimed to render psychosocial care and to refer clients to social services and mental health professionals. Such an affirmative attitude is a good opportunity to review and enhance capacities for providing psychosocial services. It should be noted, however, that the study did not include information on the nature of such services, nor on the extent of their effectiveness. There are ongoing efforts to disseminate information and train legal and health professionals within both government and non-government sectors on documentation and management of survivors of violence. However, the study observed that these training programmes are not well coordinated and are lacking in standardization and proper accreditation.

It can also be concluded from the study that safety measures are inadequate, both in the capital city and the provinces. This raises the issue of what should be the minimum requirements for opening a facility, considering that victim and caregiver safety is a responsibility of the agency/institution tasked with rendering medico-legal services.

The existence of a sufficient number of progressive and responsive legal frameworks indicates that the Philippines has the basic ingredients for a process that can lead to the formulation of a standardized national protocol for preventive and rehabilitative programmes on sexual violence. There is, however, a need to enhance interaction and coordination among the different initiatives and to move towards standardization and sustained monitoring. To this end, the process of designing a national protocol is deemed to be the most important mechanism. Such a process should:

- consider international and national frameworks and standards;
- elaborate various medical and legal interfaces and issues related to sexual violence and its prevention; and
- manage and build consensus on minimum standards, procedures and indicators.

While laws related to sexual violence are provided for in the legal system, the study noted that there is a huge gap between those provisions and actual implementation. That gap consists of a lack of a feedback mechanism on client/patient and community satisfaction with the services provided, an absence of validated parameters for evaluation, and non-existence of a monitoring and assessment scheme for state compliance with legal provisions.

There is no doubt that the Philippines can be said to be ahead, among developing countries, in initiating services addressing both medical and legal concerns in the care of female and child survivors of violence. What seems to be lacking is a process to ensure the accountability and sustainability of those services. To this end, it is suggested that stakeholders address the following issues:

- development of a professionally competent human resource pool;
- standardization of professional practice codes, with penalties for malpractice;
- creation of regulatory and certifying boards;
- formulation of requirements for continued accreditation;
- provision of continuing medical and legal education;
- development of systems and structures for ensuring standardized and adequate services and training, as well as strict adherence to rules and regulations at all levels;
- creation of a national council that is multidisciplinary and multisectoral in nature to direct and coordinate policy and advocacy on both preventive and restorative levels, as well as set standards, and will monitor implementation within the devolved structure of relevant government agencies; and
- making adequate logistical support available.